Heali

"Among all natural healing n......s, flower remedies often deserve more modern recognition for their gentle and sensuous qualities, as they provide a safe and effective treatment option that is largely free of hazardous side effects. Gudrun Penselin has created a comprehensive and insightful work on the inherent healing qualities of Bach Flowers in *Healing Spirituality: A Practical Guide to Understanding and Working with Bach Flowers.* Flush with historical insight, practical guidance and a thorough understanding of the vibrational healing powers of Bach Flowers, this book is a must-read for both beginners in the field as well as experts, who will benefit from an enriched understanding of remedial flower therapies."

—**STEVEN K. H. AUNG,** CM AOE MD PhD FAAFP
Clinical Professor, Faculty of Medicine and Dentistry,
Adjunct Professor, Faculties of Extension, Pharmacy & Pharmaceutical
Sciences and Rehabilitation Medicine and School of Public Health
University of Alberta, Edmonton, Alberta, Canada

"Gudrun's work, *Healing Spirituality,* is a loving exploration of the magnificent findings of Dr. Bach. Through decades of research, clinical practice, as well as, intuitive guidance she has brought together a comprehensive handbook that is an inspiring blend of Gudrun's contemporary approach, Dr. Bach's original work and accessible how-to use materials. Written for practitioners, enthusiasts and the curious. This is no doubt the most significant compendium I have had the pleasure to read."

—**PAULA MARIE SKALNEK**, Clinical Herbal Therapist

"Gudrun has been a healer, a support and a teacher for many years in her alternative health practice. She has a broad spectrum of knowledge balanced by respect and a deep intuitive sense of people's needs. I was introduced to the Bach Flower Cards and Bach Flower Essences as part of my treatment process. I have found both to be a source of soul strengthening insight and a path to more direct healing. I am very excited by Gudrun's new book which will allow more people exposure to this timeless and effective method of healing and personal growth."

—**KATHY ANDERSEN,** M.Sc.
Registered Clinical Psychologist
in Alberta for 35 years, recently retired

ALSO BY GUDRUN PENSELIN

Bach Flowers Unfolding
(A set of cards and a booklet with instructions
on how to use Bach Flower Remedies)

*Herbal Pharmacy for Everyone – A Step-by-Step Guide to
Creating Your Own Herbal Preparations*
(Instructional DVD with subtitles in English,
French, Spanish and German)

HEALING
SPIRITUALITY

A Practical
Guide to
Understanding
and Working
with
BACH
FLOWERS

GUDRUN PENSELIN, M.ED.

Rainbow Healing Publishing
R.R.#1, Site 1, Box 11
Wembley, AB
Canada
www.rainbowhealing.ca

ISBN 978-0-9684108-2-0

First edition 2016

Designed by AuthorSupport.com

Original art by Kay Marie Enns

Library and Archives of Canada Cataloguing in Publication is available upon request.

I dedicate this book to Mother Earth, the children of this Earth, who are our future, and in particular, to my granddaughter Vera, who brings hope and light with her joyful spirit for the healing of this planet and humankind.

"The flowers of tomorrow are in the seeds of today."

AUTHOR UNKNOWN

CONTENTS

Acknowledgements

_____

*"The action of these remedies is to raise our vibrations and
open up our channels for the reception of our Spiritual
Self, to flood our natures with the particular Virtue we
need, and wash out from us the fault which is causing
harm. They are able like beautiful music, or any gloriously
uplifting thing which gives us inspiration, to raise our very
natures, and bring us nearer to our Souls: and by that
very act, to bring us peace, and relieve our sufferings."*

—Edward Bach

I thank the inner voice that has guided me along my journey
in life. It has been an infinite source of inspiration, strength,
courage and hope, guiding me in my endeavours to support the
Earth and humankind on their path to healing. I feel blessed and
am grateful for the clarity it has given me about my purpose in life.

I am eternally grateful for the bounty and beauty of the world
of plants and all its life giving qualities, and how it continues to

provide for us in an unequalled example of unconditional Love. Thanks to the willingness of the plants to share their medicine and spirit freely I have received great support and insight from them.

Thank you to my parents who raised us in a loving environment, forever encouraging us to follow our dreams. Without their caring support and guidance in the past I would not be where I am today. They instilled in me the importance of persevering and forever following my path in life regardless of opposition or challenges along the way.

My husband, Franz, and my children Oliver, Yana-Lee and Lena, who have been on my side with understanding, support and encouragement, thank you. Oliver, Yana-Lee and Lena, you are my greatest gifts and I watch in amazement as you strive to make a positive difference in this world. My granddaughter Vera, who elicits a smile and happiness in everyone and makes difficult moments melt away bringing back sunshine into the heart.

Thank you to all my friends, teachers, clients and students. You continuously inspire me and I owe much of my learning to each one of you. Thank you to all those who, knowingly or unknowingly, contributed to my work.

No work would be accomplished without a team of people working "behind the scenes" throughout the process of creation. A special heartfelt thank you to Lana who has been my chief editor; we spent many days together, and hours on the phone, combing through the material. Thank you Lana!

Thank you, Kathy, for taking time out of your demanding schedule to provide valuable feedback and Catherine, for supporting me in the final stages up to the last minute. Thank you for being here for me with such encouraging and kind support. Thank you, Martha, for sharing your expertise, resources and friendly advice, guiding me step by step through the uncharted territory of writing and publishing a book. Thank you to every one of you for making it so easy to work with you. A special thank you to Donna Marie who supported me as a friend with her invaluable insights.

Gudrun Penselin, M.Ed., M. Phys. Ed.
Clinical Herbal Therapist
Bach Flower Practitioner

PREFACE

HEALING SPIRITUALITY was written as an expansion and continuation of *Bach Flowers Unfolding*. Bach Flower essences are plant medicines that provide support and healing through addressing a person's mental states and emotions. Bach Flowers, through their vibrational frequencies, have the ability to open and enhance our communication with our Higher Self, and in this way encourage healing in all aspects – emotional, spiritual, mental and physical. The ultimate goal is to free ourselves of limitations that hold us back from fulfilling our purpose in life.

The book serves as a practical guide and working tool for the implementation of Bach Flowers into a person's daily life. Edward Bach's original work has been carefully preserved, but the increase in the vibrational frequencies of the Earth affects the information and healing potential brought forth by the Bach Flowers. Therefore, the information relating to the 38 Bach Flowers plus the Rescue Remedy has been adjusted to the changes occurring on the planet at this time.

Please note: For the benefit of the general flow when reading the book I use, where applicable, either *he* or *she*, implying both.

INTRODUCTION

---

*"Serving through love in perfect freedom in
our own way is success, is health."*

—EDWARD BACH

HEALING SPIRITUALITY is the result of my personal journey which has been one of many discoveries and realizations. Again and again I have wondered why I have felt so compelled to complete this work. Many times I have played with the idea of abandoning this project, wanting to believe that I could simplify my life by shifting my entire focus to my growing family with grandchildren and a thriving complementary health practice; there seemed to be more than enough to fulfill me. Regardless of how hard I wanted to change course, I knew deep down in my heart that advancing Edward Bach's information to the higher vibrational frequencies of the planet is what I must do in order to follow the mission of my Soul – to serve humanity and Mother Earth.

*"Our soul (the still small voice, God's own voice) speaks
to us through our intuition, our instincts, our desires,
ideals, our ordinary likes and dislikes; in whichever
way it is easiest for us individually to hear."*

—EDWARD BACH

For me the voice that Edward Bach refers to is best described as a sense of inner knowing. Not listening to it would certainly put fewer demands on my busy schedule, but would ultimately result in unhappiness, possibly leading to undesirable health challenges. So I have decided to travel my journey with joy in my heart and I am happy to share with you HEALING SPIRITUALITY.

HEALING SPIRITUALITY is an expansion and continuation of my previous publication, *Bach Flowers Unfolding*. *Bach Flowers Unfolding* is a deck of cards, one for each flower, with artwork and channeled text. The essence of Edward Bach's original work has been carefully preserved. The deck of cards serves as a unique and innovative tool for working with the Bach Flowers. Over the years it has provided support and healing to many who have looked for guidance on their journey. Depending on circumstances and the individual, working with the cards alone, especially in the initial stages, will often bring more profound healing than taking the actual remedies. Numerous testimonials and thank you letters, as well as my first hand observations when teaching classes, have proven this to be true time and time again.

As the vibrational frequencies of the Earth have been increasing steadily, bringing life to a dimension of enlightened awareness, the need once again arises to adjust the information brought forth by the Bach Flowers. The revised information ensures that the Bach Flowers continue to serve all life forms on the planet in moving forward and living a life in accordance with their Soul purpose.

I have created this work under Dr. Bach's spiritual guidance as well as through direct intuitive communication with the spirit of the Bach Flowers, adjusting the information forward to harmonize with the changing vibrational frequencies of the Earth. In order to be able to align with the Earth our physical bodies also need to move into higher frequencies. Once our frequencies work in unison our lives will be enriched, communication with spirit will flow more easily and clearly and we will find our way back to the values that truly matter, including re-connecting to our Mother, the Earth. As a result, we will be moving towards inner peace and happiness, healing ourselves and the planet.

My wish for you is that HEALING SPIRITUALITY deepens your understanding of this marvelous and miraculous system of healing and at the same time serves as a self-help guide for working with Bach Flowers. May their gentle yet powerful spirit come alive for you and within you. I encourage you to allow the essence of the Bach Flowers to support and guide you on your healing journey to wholeness, synchronized balance and the Light. Peace on Earth for all is possible as a result of healing spirituality.

CHAPTER 1

My Personal Journey and Experience with Bach Flowers

*"I see Gudrun as a healer and friend to those around
her and the Earth itself, and am constantly inspired
to strengthen my own commitment to living a life
based in Love, and the singular dedication to the
much needed healing of this Earth and its people."*

—**LANA ROBINSON,** B.A. (Psychology and Political
Science); Presiding Clerk of Canadian Friends Service
Committee (CFSC); Community Health Organizer

I was born and raised in Germany and like so many children back
then we played outside much of the time. Preventative health
in the form of healthy lifestyle choices was an integral part of
my upbringing.

My parents were very caring, supportive and tolerant but at the
same time had high expectations, which focused on the intellect
and academic achievements. Even though these expectations were

not necessarily expressed verbally, they were always present in a subtle way, something my parents were probably not even aware of themselves. This mindset profoundly influenced me in a challenging way because I live my life first and foremost through my heart where emotions and feelings are the guiding stars in contrast to the intellect. As a result, my life has been dominated for many years by feelings of never being good enough, never being able to accomplish anything to my personal satisfaction and a lack of self-worth. After my discovery of the Bach Flowers almost 30 years ago, the essence of the flower from the *Pine* tree became my best friend and for many years helped me to overcome these feelings of inadequacy.

I am often asked when and how I got involved with Bach Flowers. The only answer I have is that I cannot remember. I know I was already running my own practice as a complementary health practitioner and that I began acquiring individual remedies for use with clients and my family. Eventually I ordered a complete kit with all 38 individual flower essences plus the *Rescue Remedy*. It remains a mystery how, or by whom, I was introduced to this marvelous and miraculous form of vibrational healing. However, the truly significant fact is that Edward Bach's work resonated deeply with me from the very beginning. Ever since my initial introduction, Bach Flowers have been an integral part of my life–as part of my practice with clients, with my family, friends and of course myself. Bach Flowers serve us in all walks of life and in all aspects – spiritual, emotional, mental and physical. To me they are like best friends who are always here to lend a helping hand as support in daily life, in a crisis, when I am seeking an answer to a question or for direction in my life.

In my practice I integrate Bach Flower therapy as an adjunct to any other healing modality in order to enhance the healing process. Regardless of which form or combination of therapy is being applied (reflexology, herbal medicine, light and colour therapy, iridology, sclerology, energy medicine etc.) Bach Flowers are always a valuable addition to the program of holistic wellness. Staying true to Edward Bach's philosophy of making his system of healing affordable to all, my clients receive their treatment bottles free of charge, with unlimited refills.

After many years of experience with the Bach Flowers I was spiritually guided to develop *Bach Flowers Unfolding*. This deck of cards gives a detailed description about the respective flower essence in regard to the present state of mind and emotional circumstances a person is experiencing as well as the potentially transformed state. Exquisite full colour illustrations enhance the text. It is an innovative, unique and exciting publication about the Bach Flowers, revealing new levels of information. The cards themselves carry the essence of the Bach Flowers, providing support and healing due to the high vibrational frequencies of the text as well as the art, and the intent underlying the creation of this work.

When I travel I always carry a deck of cards with me as support in case I need it. They have proven to be a true life saver for me in challenging situations.

In my teenage years I developed a strong desire to travel to India. I decided to spend half a year there after completing high school and before entering university. During my travels I was blessed to spend some time with Mother Teresa in Calcutta, primarily helping with orphaned infants. Mother Teresa worked with the heart and Soul of people, with compassion and non-judgment. "*If you judge people, you have no time to love them.*" (Mother Teresa) Both Mother Teresa and Edward Bach had the strong desire to ease suffering in this world and found their own unique ways to fulfill their mission in life. Their legacies, as well as their words and wisdom, continue to influence people's lives worldwide. My time in India, my work with Mother Teresa and my experiences with the Bach Flowers, changed my life forever and I continue to be inspired to live my life in service to the Earth and its people.

In 1981 I emigrated to Canada where I have focused my professional education on complementary medicine. For over 30 years I have been running a successful practice in Grande Prairie, Alberta. Over the years I have helped thousands of people through my teachings and practice by using a holistic approach to wellness, always considering all aspects of our being – emotional, spiritual, physical and mental.

My joy and passion is to encourage others on their healing journey and support them in unfolding to their full potential. I am filled with gratitude when I watch my clients and students leave my office feeling empowered and stronger, filled with hope and carrying a big smile on their face.

I offer workshops in all the healing arts that I utilize in my practice. My classes are experiential and interactive, with a focus on practicality and fun. Due to the nature of the workshops and my teaching style students commonly experience some form of healing from my courses. One of my favorite classes includes teaching students how to connect to plant spirit.

Ever since I can remember I have had great respect for traditional medicine from other cultures. Their understanding of and connection to the land has always impressed and intrigued me. Over the past few years my dream to learn from traditional healers has been fulfilled. I have been fortunate to be able to spend time with healers in Central and South America and experience some of their practices including one of my favourites, the temazcal (sweatlodge).

I look on the Earth as our Mother who provides for us with unconditional love regardless of the abuse by the human race. In my practice and teachings I re-awaken in people this awareness and the connection to the Earth, a prerequisite for the healing of the planet and humankind. Due to my own strong connection with the Earth I am able to connect and communicate with plant spirit, allowing me to channel the information directly from the Bach Flowers under the guiding light of Edward Bach. I consider myself blessed beyond measure to be conscious of my mission in life – something I owe in part to the Bach Flowers. Thank you, Dr. Edward Bach!

> *"There are saints at the factory bench and in the stokehold of a ship as well as among the dignitaries of religious orders. Not one of us upon this earth is being asked to do more than is within his power to perform, and if we strive to obtain the best within us, ever guided by our Higher Self, health and happiness is a possibility for each one."*
>
> **—EDWARD BACH**

CHAPTER 2

Bach Flowers — A System of Vibrational Healing

*"... those beautiful remedies, which have been Divinely
enriched with healing powers, will be administered, to open
up those channels to admit more of the light of the Soul,
that the patient may be flooded with healing virtue. They
cure not by attacking disease, but by flooding our bodies
with the beautiful vibrations of our Higher Nature, in the
presence of which disease melts as snow in the sunshine."*

—EDWARD BACH

With the creation of the flower essences known as Bach Flowers, Edward Bach developed a system of vibrational healing that continues to spread worldwide, changing the lives of more and more people. He planted the seeds over 80 years ago that give hope, peace, courage, joy, health, happiness and so much more to humankind, the animal and plant kingdoms and indeed the entire planet.

BACH FLOWERS EXPLAINED

*"These plants are there to extend a helping hand to man in
those dark hours of forgetfulness, when he loses sight of divinity,
and allows the cloud of fear or pain to obscure his vision."*

—EDWARD BACH

Bach Flowers are flower essences made from blooms, buds, young leaves and flowering twigs of plants and trees except for one remedy, *Rock Water,* which originates from spring water. The system was developed by Edward Bach and includes 38 individual essences plus one combination of five different Bach Flowers which he named the *Rescue Remedy*. Edward Bach divided the system into seven main categories, each addressing one major mental state.

An essence can be described as the energetic imprint of a flower, leaf, rock, crystal etc. which has been transferred into and absorbed by water. The flower essences are non-toxic herbal preparations that affect all levels of our being, with the primary focus being a person's mental and emotional states as well as their spiritual well-being. Since the health of our physical body is closely related to our emotions, mental outlook and spirit, the body is often able to create physical balance once harmony is being achieved in the other three aspects.

Edward Bach, a medical doctor from England, developed this system of healing in the years between 1930 to 1936. He believed that physical disease (dis-ease) was primarily the result of imbalances in our mind and emotions. In his search to find a method of healing as an alternative to modern medicine he discovered the power of plants. He realized that each plant holds its own unique signature and personality.

When prepared in a specific way and taken at the right time, these plants assist any living organism to resolve the imbalances which cause distress and dis-ease to physical, mental, emotional and spiritual well-being. The Bach Flower essences open channels of communication to our Higher Self, encouraging us to recognize who we are and why we are here on this Earth. Ultimately they support and guide us in freeing ourselves of any limitations that might hold us back from living our lives to the fullest and in accordance with our Soul essence.

BACH FLOWER ESSENCES VERSUS HOMEOPATHY

"True hate may be conquered by a greater hate, but it can only be cured by love, cruelty may be prevented by a greater cruelty, but only eliminated when the qualities of sympathy and pity have developed, one fear may be lost and forgotten in the presence of a greater fear, but the real cure of fear is perfect courage."
—**EDWARD BACH**

People commonly assume that Bach Flower essences are the same as homeopathic preparations; however, this belief is incorrect. Edward Bach himself was very familiar with Samuel Hahnemann, the founder of homeopathy, and had great respect for him and his work. Bach considered the system of healing with Bach Flower essences as an advancement of homeopathy.

"Hahnemann made a great advance and carried us a long way along the road, but he had only the length of one life in which

to work, and it is for us to continue his researches where he left
off, to add more to the structure of perfect healing of which he
laid the foundation, and so worthily began the building."

—EDWARD BACH

Both homeopathy and Bach Flower essences belong to a larger category of healing defined as energy medicine or vibrational healing, (see below for details) but there are distinct differences between the two. The differences lie in the underlying principle, the method of preparation and the way a remedy is chosen.

Homeopathy is based on the doctrine that "like cures like" which means that a substance that can cause symptoms of dis-ease in a healthy person can cure similar symptoms in a sick individual. Substances chosen for treatment are the ones that produce symptoms matching the condition of the client.

Instead, Bach Flower essences work with the positive virtue that is desirable to attain. Bach believed that this would create a free flowing connection to a person's Higher Self and as a result, encourage the individual to become aware of their situation and allow them to make more conscious choices. Therefore, rather than adding more darkness to darkness in order to create light, Bach Flower essences create light by adding light. If a person is filled with fear the Bach Flower essence applied may give courage to overcome the fear. Specifics depend of course on the individual and circumstances.

"And so in true healing, and so in spiritual advancement, we
must always seek good to drive out evil, love to conquer hate,
and light to dispel darkness. Thus must we avoid all poisons,
all harmful things, and use only the beneficent and beautiful."

—EDWARD BACH

Unlike homeopathy, the choice of a Bach Flower essence is solely based on emotional and mental aspects without taking the physical into consideration. The ultimate goal is to bring us closer to our Soul because *"Health depends on being in harmony with our souls."* (Edward Bach)

Bach Flowers are made from flowers and buds of flowering plants and trees (with the exception of *Rock Water*). In comparison, the homeopathic mother tincture is prepared by extracting properties from various plant materials such as roots, barks, flowers etc. as well as minerals and stones, animal and human substances. The materials used in homeopathic remedies are then macerated in alcohol for several weeks. The process involves continuous dilutions which are potentiated through a specific rhythmic method known as trituration. The entire process takes place indoors.

On the other hand, Bach Flower essences are prepared outside with all the elements of nature involved. Their essence or distinctive imprint is imparted into spring water for just several hours before creating the mother tincture. The properties are only extracted from the flowering parts and when the flowers are at their peak time of blossoming.

NOTE: At times people confuse Bach Flowers with aromatherapy– another form of vibrational medicine. Aromatherapy works with the volatile oils of plant material that are characterized by specific smells which, when absorbed by the body, will trigger a certain response. Bach Flower essences do not work through the sense of smell.

HOW BACH FLOWERS WORK THROUGH VIBRATIONAL HEALING

"The action of these remedies is to raise our vibrations and open up our channels for the reception of our Spiritual

Self, to flood our natures with the particular Virtue we need, and wash out from us the fault which is causing harm. They are able like beautiful music, or any gloriously uplifting thing which gives us inspiration, to raise our very natures, and bring us nearer to our Souls: and by that very act, to bring us peace, and relieve our sufferings."

—EDWARD BACH

Bach Flower essences work in many ways and on various levels. Even though Edward Bach emphasized that the use of this healing system should be kept *"free from science, free from theories, for everything in nature is simple",* curiosity and the desire of the human mind to understand has driven people to explore why Bach Flowers work the way they do.

Their healing potential can best be described as the result of vibrational healing, a term that has become more widely used and accepted over the past years and is seen by some as the medicine of the future. Vibrational medicine or energy medicine is based on the scientific principle that all matter vibrates to a precise frequency and that by using resonant vibration, balance of matter can be restored. This is illustrated by Ernst Chladni's discovery in 1786. Chladni was a German physicist and musician who demonstrated that iron shavings placed on a plate or membrane will form geometric patterns when using a tone generator to cause the plate to vibrate. As the pitch increases the frequencies, the geometric patterns will become more complex.

Every cell, every organism is characterized by its own unique vibrational frequencies. For optimal health, which includes all aspects – physical, mental, emotional and spiritual – the cells in our body need to vibrate in harmony with each other and in unison with the Earth, our spirit and our Soul. Any discord or imbalance in these frequencies can lead to experiences of disharmony and stress. Depending on the severity, the duration and our inherent individual make-up, this imbalance manifests in different ways. The more sensitive person and the one who is more in-tune with all aspects of their being will be aware of even subtle changes in their energies. Someone else who is less sensitive, has a stronger constitution or has learned to disassociate themselves from their emotions will not be aware of subtle changes. As a result, they are not as quick to make necessary adjustments in their lives in order to restore balance and avoid major downfalls as time passes.

Vibrational healing or energy medicine is a phenomenon that cannot be discredited. We cannot see the wind yet we can feel it and know it is there. We cannot see the sounds of nature or any music being created, but we can hear it and know that it is real. Bach Flower essences work under the same principle. Their effect and healing potential are not tangible yet their spirit touches us on deep levels with their harmonizing effect.

There are many forms of vibrational medicine, Bach Flower essences are only one of them. It is noteworthy that the essences of Bach Flowers, and plants in general, include more than one aspect of vibrational healing. In addition to the spirit essence of the flowers, they also bring forth frequencies of colour, light and sound. All of these are different forms of energy medicine. Every flower creates its own song due to vibrational frequencies unique to it. I have been fortunate to have heard these voices of nature and capture them on a video.

Vibrational healing with Bach Flower essences affects deep levels of consciousness, shifting emotions, stimulating one's own healing potential, providing support to the physical body and ultimately restoring balance and bringing us closer to our Soul.

CHAPTER 3

Edward Bach

*"Every kindly smile, every kindly thought and action;
every deed done for love or sympathy or compassion of
others proves that there is something greater within us
than what we see. That we carry a Spark of the Divine,
that within us resides a Vital and Immortal principle."*

—EDWARD BACH

Edward Bach was born in Moseley, near Birmingham, England on September 24, 1886, and passed on November 27, 1936 at the age of 50. His ancestry was Welsh and he was the first of three children in a family of two boys and one girl. Bach was a very delicate baby requiring special care for the first few years of his life. As he got older he gained strength and was able to live a normal life. From a very young age he felt compassion for any living creatures that were suffering and he had the desire to ease their pain. This and his love for nature were the foundations of his personality and of his search for a simple and effective form of healing.

"This love of Wales drew Edward Bach to her (nature) again
and again. When he was a schoolboy he would spend his
holidays tramping through the Welsh villages and over the
mountains, sleeping each night where he could, happy in the
company of his friends the birds and trees and wild flowers,
for his love of Nature showed itself at a very young age."*

—NORA WEEKS

At the age of 16, upon completion of his schooling, he
worked at his father's brass foundry for three years before
entering medical school in 1907. He worked in all departments
of the company; when working in sales his good heart made him
promise prices to customers that were impossible to meet. He
disliked the regular hours and spending most of his time indoors.
However, those three years gave him the opportunity to spend
time observing people which would lay part of the foundation
of his later work.

In 1917 at the age of 31 he suffered a severe hemorrhage as a
result of a malignant tumor. He was given only three months to
live. His deep longing to find a system of healing that met his ideas
and ideals gave him the strength to overcome this serious illness
and continue work on his life's mission. He lived 19 more years.
His recovery led him to the conclusion that a person's state of
mind was the key to understanding health and dis-ease and *"that
an absorbing interest, a great love, a definite purpose in life was the
deciding factor of a man's happiness on earth."* (Nora Weeks)

Bach's desire to support humankind and ease suffering led
him to study medicine and become a doctor and bacteriologist. Even at that time he was convinced that a simpler form of

---
*   Author's note

healing could be found but he knew that he needed to study medicine first.

Throughout his education and practice as a medical doctor he felt that practical experience and acute observation of patients and people in general were much more important than studying from books. Indeed, he was known to have said on being presented with his medical degrees: *"It will take me five years to forget all I have been taught."* Bach considered his intuition and practical experience to be his most valuable teachers in life.

Bach was driven to find a form of medicine that was gentle, painless, benign and effective in providing true and long-lasting healing. He also wanted to by-pass often painful and lengthy medical diagnostic procedures. In his search for such a system he soon realized that the success of a treatment was strongly influenced by the personality of the individual. Therefore, treating the person as a whole, rather than treating the dis-ease and its symptoms alone, was required if true healing should occur. Bach considered physical illness a great opportunity to heal the mind and the emotions, resulting in a deepened connection to our own Soul and the Divine.

Guided by his strong connection to spirit he eventually discovered the healing powers of plants and developed this incredible system of vibrational medicine known today as the Bach Flowers.

HIS PERSONALITY

"Thus every personality we meet in life, whether mother, husband, child, stranger or friend, becomes a fellow-traveller, and any of them may be greater or smaller than ourselves as regards spiritual development; but all of us are members of a

*common brotherhood and part of a great community making
the same journey with the same glorious end in view."*

—EDWARD BACH

Edward Bach's personality has been described as mischievous, full of vitality, yet quiet and at times meditative. He enjoyed being among people of all walks of life. Bach had a very compassionate nature; he was humble, well liked, positive and had a great sense of humor. However, his strong determination and intense character made it difficult for some to relate to him. His highly evolved spirit allowed him to be conscious of his important purpose in life from an early age.

Bach's belief in the importance of always listening to his Higher Self and following his Soul's guidance were contributing factors to his independent personality. These attributes gave him the courage and conviction to pursue his purpose in life; they were the driving force behind many of his actions and decisions.

Bach was a genius with exceptional intellectual and creative powers and was gifted with a highly developed intuitive sense as well as the innate ability to heal.

*"So strongly was he guided by inspiration that
anything interfering with intuitive action not only
gave him a sense of dissatisfaction and unfulfillment,
but left him physically exhausted and ill."*

—NORA WEEKS

HIS DREAMS

"Everything about the hospital of the future will be
uplifting and beautiful, so that the patient will seek that
refuge, not only to be relieved of his malady, but also to
develop the desire to live a life more in harmony with the
dictates of his Soul than had been previously done."

—Edward Bach

Early on in his life Bach dreamed of becoming a medical doctor as well as finding a simple form of healing for curing all diseases. During his medical career, he became increasingly dissatisfied with conventional medicine and his experiences as a medical doctor led him to believe that there must be a system of healing that provided true healing in all aspects of life – emotional, mental, spiritual and physical. His dream was to find this new method; he eventually followed his calling, knowing that he would find the answer to his dream in nature, among the plants and the trees.

After Edward Bach left London in 1930 he envisioned a different medical system altogether; a system where doctors would understand people as individuals and treat them as such rather than focus on the dis-ease alone. Instead of studying lab results he imagined doctors studying human nature and supporting patients in understanding the lessons of life, in encouraging them to take responsibility for their own well-being and ultimately guiding them to a life lived in harmony with their Soul. He imagined the hospital of the future as a sanctuary where people would find peace, hope, joy and faith. Bach also imagined being able to use his hands for healing; he eventually discovered that he was granted this gift as well.

HIS PROFESSIONAL CAREER

*"Life to him was continuous; an unbroken stream,
uninterrupted by what we call death, which merely heralded
a change of conditions, and he was convinced that some
work could only be done under earthly conditions, whilst
spiritual conditions were necessary for certain works."*

—EDWARD BACH

Edward Bach believed that in order to find the truth about
dis-ease and healing he had to study medicine first. In 1907
Edward Bach entered Birmingham University where he began
his medical training. Later he moved to London to continue his
studies at the University College Hospital. Bach graduated in
1912 with the Conjunct Diploma of MRCS (Member of the
Royal College of Surgeons) and LRCP (Licentiate of the Royal
College of Physicians). In 1913 he was awarded additional
degrees, MB (*Medicinae Baccalaureus*, Bachelor of Medicine)
and BS (Bachelor of Science). Bach had *"little use for accepted
theories until he had proven them for himself. Practical experience and observation were to him the only true way of learning."*
(Nora Weeks)

From 1912 to 1930 Edward Bach held various posts including
House Surgeon and Head of the Emergency Department at the
University College Hospital, and assistant in the Department of
Bacteriology and Immunology. In 1913 he began his research into
vaccines, eventually preparing them from intestinal bacteria. This
work brought him international acclaim.

In 1918 a flu epidemic broke out in the trenches among the
soldiers fighting in the first World War; the flu spread quickly

to the home countries of the soldiers including England, killing millions. During that time Bach was unofficially allowed to treat soldiers with these vaccines which saved thousands of lives.

> *"The vaccines he prepared from intestinal bacteria were being more and more used in the treatment of chronic disease, and with such excellent results that the method was adopted generally by the medical profession."*
>
> **—NORA WEEKS**

His work at the London Homeopathic Hospital as bacteriologist and pathologist put him in touch with homeopathy and the work of Samuel Hahnemann. The underlying principle of homeopathy, to treat the patient and not the dis-ease, correlated with Bach's observations that each case needed individual consideration. Bach began to prepare the vaccines by the homeopathic methods which were given orally instead of being injected. These vaccines are still known today as the seven Bach nosodes.

Bach practiced medicine for over 20 years in London in his private practice in Harley Street while also working in his laboratory, continuing relentlessly his research into finding a cure for all dis-ease. His practice and fame were growing steadily with the success of his work.

Bach disliked the busy city life of London, longing for the peace and quiet of the countryside and being surrounded by his friends of nature. He suppressed this desire, not even visiting nearby parks of London because he was afraid that this would distract him from his research and the possibility of finding the new method of healing. Therefore, from 1912 to 1930 he rarely left London.

*"It is ironic that the very love of nature that he
was trying to suppress within himself would
later lead him to the remedies he sought."*

(VIDEO: THE LIGHT THAT NEVER GOES OUT)

In 1924 Bach presented a paper entitled *Intestinal Toxaemia
in its Relation to Cancer* at the British Homeopathic Congress in
London. In this work he suggests that a diet of raw foods, fruits,
nuts, cereals and vegetables reduces the amount of toxins produced
in the intestines. This type of diet combined with his vaccines did
not focus on the local treatment of the cancer. Bach realized that
the beneficial effect on the cancer patients was primarily the result
of general improvements of their health.

In September of 1928 Bach felt a sudden urge to go to Wales;
following his intuition he left his practice in London and jour-
neyed to Wales. Here he found the first two of the 38 Bach
Flowers, *Impatiens* and *Mimulus*. Upon his return to London
he prepared these two flowers using the homeopathic method.
When prescribing *Impatiens* and *Mimulus* to patients according
to their personality, his patients would experience remarkable
results. Later that year he added *Clematis* to his repertoire. The
discovery of these three Bach Flower remedies signaled the beginning of a new stage in his life.

The same year Bach attended a dinner where he spent much of
the time observing the other guests when it suddenly occurred to
him that all of humanity consisted of a definite number of groups
of personality types. He later realized that the individuals of each
group would not necessarily contract the same dis-ease but their
reaction to disease was the same. This observation would become
one of the fundamental principles of the Bach Flower system.

In 1930 Bach abandoned the homeopathic way of preparing

the Bach Flower essences and developed the sun and boiling methods. See Chapter 15, *Instructions for Creating Bach Flower Essences,* for details. From this time on Bach felt more than ever in tune with his spirituality and intuitive senses. He left conventional medicine in search of a new system of healing.

Bach's colleagues and friends were surprised by his decision because they considered him a leader in scientific research and were certain that he would further advance the field of medicine through new discoveries. Except for one doctor, Dr. John H. Clarke, Bach's colleagues could not comprehend why he set out to follow his ideals and leave his medical career behind. Dr. Clarke encouraged Bach the evening before he left London with the following words:

> *"My lad, forget all you have learnt, forget the past*
> *and go ahead. You will find what you are seeking,*
> *and when you have found it I will welcome you back*
> *and give you my support. ... may I live to see the day*
> *that you return for I know what you find will bring*
> *great joy and comfort to those for whom we, at present,*
> *can do so little. I shall be prepared to give my work*
> *to the flames, and set up instead as a practitioner*
> *of the new and better medicine you will find."*
>
> **—NORA WEEKS**

Bach divided his lucrative practice in London between his medical friends and closed down his laboratory, following his calling to return to nature.

> *"He made a large bonfire of all the pamphlets and*
> *papers he had written on his former work, and*

*smashed syringes and vaccine bottles, throwing
their contents down the laboratory sink."*

—NORA WEEKS

From 1930 to 1936 Bach discovered all 38 Bach Flowers in the fields, the meadows, along the streams and in the mountains of England and Wales. For further details, see Chapter 6, *Discovery of the Bach Flowers.*

Bach considered his new system of healing a gift of the Divine and not a human creation. He believed that the 38 Bach Flowers plus the *Rescue Remedy* comprise a system that is complete within itself not requiring the addition of any other remedies.

Bach was content with his final work because he felt his purpose in life had been fulfilled. Bach Flower remedies are simple to use and can be used by anyone. They affirm that everyone has the power to heal, and encourage each one of us to understand who we are, listen to our Higher Self and take charge of our own destiny by following our Soul's guidance. We are all healers.

In order to avoid confusion Bach believed that it was best to keep only his final research findings. As was his custom he destroyed in a bonfire all his notes with the theories and ideas leading up to the completion of the new method of healing with Bach Flowers. He felt that his book, *The Twelve Healers and Other Remedies*, contained all the information required for people to apply and continue his work.

BACH'S CONTROVERSIAL RELATIONSHIP WITH THE MEDICAL COMMUNITY

Edward Bach drew a lot of criticism from the establishment in the medical system. From 1932 to 1936 he received several warnings from the General Medical Council (the body with the legal responsibility for regulating the medical profession in the UK) regarding some small advertisements he placed in newspapers and for using unqualified assistants. However, he believed in the benefit of his work for all and in 1936, after being threatened by the General Medical Council once again to be taken off the Medical Register, he replied with the following letter.

Wellsprings, Sotwell, Wallingford, BERKS.

January 8, 1936

To the President of the Medical Council.

Dear Sir,

Having received the notification of the Council concerning working with unqualified assistants, it is only honourable to inform you that I am working with several, and shall continue to do so.

As I have previously informed the Council, I consider it the duty and privilege of any physician to teach the sick and others how to heal themselves. I leave it entirely to your discretion as to the course you take.

Having proved that the Herbs of the field are so simple to use and so wonderfully effective in their healing powers, I deserted Orthodox medicine.

Registered medical address.

Berryfields, Park Lane, Ashstead, Surrey.

CHAPTER 4

Edward Bach's Beliefs and Philosophy of Life And Healing

*"Let us develop our individuality that we may obtain
complete freedom to serve the Divinity within ourselves,
and that Divinity alone, and give unto all others their
absolute freedom, and serve them as much as lies within
our power, according to the dictates of our Souls, ever
remembering that as our own liberty increases, so grows
our freedom and ability to serve our fellow-men."*

—EDWARD BACH

Edward Bach was a remarkable individual who had deep insights into the nature of human beings and life in general. The few original writings still available today are evidence of his incredible mind and understanding and are as valid today, and possibly even more important now, as they were during his life time.

Bach believed that healing is of Divine origin and is above all materialistic things and laws. Healing must come from within. He considered materialism as darkness and disagreed with the notion that dis-ease is of purely materialistic nature and could be cured with materialistic means alone.

According to Bach, greed was one of the greatest faults of mankind and therefore reason for dis-ease. He not only considered this in terms of greed for wealth or other worldly things but felt that the worst kind of greed is the desire to influence and control the life of another individual.

> *"The moment that we ourselves have given complete liberty to all around us, when we no longer expect anything from anyone, when our only thought is to give and give and never to take, that moment shall we find that we are free of all the world, our bonds will fall from us, our chains be broken, and for the first time in our lives shall we know the exquisite joy of perfect liberty. Freed from all human restraint, the willing and joyous servant of our Higher Self alone."*
>
> **—EDWARD BACH**

Health cannot be obtained "*by payment of gold*" (Edward Bach) just like the learning of skills cannot be purchased with money. Disease originates from the mental plane rather than the physical and true healing involves the creation of harmony between one's Soul, emotions, body and mind. This harmony between our spiritual and mortal self can only be achieved by one's own efforts, although we may at times be guided by an experienced teacher or friend.

Bach knew that our Mother, the Earth, was providing the clean, pure elements required for healing. He was guided by the Divine to the beautiful Bach Flowers and understood that they have been given to us for their gentle, yet powerful healing attributes and are able to open the channels to our Soul and in this way flood our being with their healing virtues by increasing our vibrational frequencies. Feelings of peace, hope, joy and faith are being brought forth.

SIMPLICITY

"SIMPLICITY is the key to all creation."

—EDWARD BACH

Simplicity was one of Bach's key principles and greatly influenced the search for and development of this new method of healing. It is this simplicity that puts the power of healing into the hands of everyone. This underlying principle was greatly emphasized throughout his writings, teachings and in his practice. No knowledge of medicine or science is required for the use of the Bach Flower essences because they address a person's state of mind, emotions and personality, disregarding entirely the symptoms or dis-ease of the physical body.

Bach wanted to convey how simple the Bach Flower system of healing is. He believed that each one of us is a healer and because of the simplicity of this new system, anyone could prescribe and treat oneself or others with the appropriate Bach Flower essences in order to restore balance – mental, emotional, spiritual and physical.

In 1936, two months before his death, Bach gave a public lecture in Wallingford, England, entitled: *Healing by Herbs – For use in every Home.* At that time, he addressed the joy the use of the Bach Flower essences could bring to anyone who desired to do something for those who were ill or in need of support. *"It gives to them the power to be healers amongst their fellows."* (Edward Bach)

During the process of our healing journey with the Bach Flowers we get a deeper sense of who we are, enabling us to take charge of our own destiny more easily.

Bach envisioned this new method of healing to be as simple as: *"I am hungry, I will go and pull a lettuce from the garden for my tea; I am frightened and ill, I will take a dose of Mimulus."*

It is not only the simplicity of actually using Bach Flowers for healing that he had longed for but at the same time the preparation of the remedies should remain free of scientific theories and complicated procedures. He developed a method for extracting the healing properties of the plants that, if desired, allows every person to create their own Bach Flower essences. Staying true to his principles Bach made all the information readily available to anyone.

Bach had the gift of using his hands for healing but he knew that this gift is not shared by everyone and that it cannot be taught or learned easily. He was delighted that healing with the Bach Flower essences places the same power of healing in the hands of all.

"Let not the simplicity of this method deter you from its use. For you will find that the further your research is advanced the greater you will realize the simplicity of all creation."

—EDWARD BACH

HEALTH AND HEALING

"Health is our heritage, our right. It is the complete and full union between soul, mind and body; and this is not difficult to attain, but one so easy and natural that many of us have overlooked it."

—EDWARD BACH

Edward Bach was a compassionate genius and pioneer driven to find a form of healing that would be painless, affordable for all and most importantly would provide true healing in contrast to suppressing symptoms and thereby driving the disease deeper into the system. His life experiences, his highly developed intuition and deep connection to nature, combined with a strong desire to ease suffering led him to develop a personal philosophy about life, health and healing.

Following are a few points outlining some of his belief system which he wrote about in his book *Heal Thyself – An Explanation of the Real Cause and Cure of Disease*. This book is one of my favorite works by him because it so clearly describes his philosophy about life and healing.

- *"Life is harmony – a state of being in tune – and that disease is discord, a condition when a part of the whole is not vibrating in unison."*
- *"The main reason for the failure of modern medical science is that it is dealing with results and not causes."*
- *"Disease will never be cured or eradicated by present materialistic methods, for the simple reason that disease in its origin is not material. What we know as disease is an ultimate result produced in the body, the end product of deep and long-acting forces, and even if material treatment alone is apparently successful this is nothing more than a temporary relief unless the real cause has been removed. The modern trend of medical science, by misinterpreting the true nature of disease and concentrating it in materialistic terms in the physical body, has enormously increased its power, firstly by distracting the thoughts of people from its true origin and hence from the effective method of attack*

and secondly, by localising it in the body, thus obscuring true hope of recovery and raising a mighty disease complex of fear, which never should have existed."

- "The knowledge of bacteria and various germs associated with disease has played havoc in the minds of tens of thousands of people, and by the dread aroused in them has in itself rendered them more susceptible of attack. While lower forms of life, such as bacteria, may play a part in or be associated with physical disease, they constitute by no means the whole truth of the problem, as can be demonstrated scientifically or by everyday occurrences."

- "So we see there are two great possible fundamental errors: disassociation between our Souls and our personalities, and cruelty or wrong to others, for this is a sin against Unity. Either of these brings conflict, which leads to disease."

- "Disease is in essence the result of conflict between Soul and Mind, and will never be eradicated except by spiritual and mental effort."

- "Disease is the result in the physical body of the resistance of the personality to the guidance of the soul."

- "...disease, though apparently so cruel, is in itself beneficent and for our good and, if rightly interpreted, it will guide us to our essential faults."

- "Disease... has for its object the bringing back of the personality to the Divine will of the Soul."

- "The real primary disease of man are such defects as pride, cruelty, hate, self-love, ignorance, instability and greed; and each of these, if considered, will be adverse to Unity."

- "...there is nothing of the nature of accident as regards disease, either in its type or in that part of the body which is affected; like all other results of energy, it follows the law of cause and effect."

- "...final and complete healing ultimately comes from within, from the Soul itself."

- "...so long as our Souls and personalities are in harmony all is joy and peace, happiness and health."

- "... that Love is the foundation of Creation, that in every living soul there is some good and that in the best of us there is some bad."

- "Love and Unity are the great foundations of our Creation, ...we ourselves are children of the Divine Love, and ... the eternal conquest of all wrong and suffering will be accomplished by means of gentleness and love."

- The disease "is only a symptom of the cause, and as the cause will manifest itself differently in nearly every individual, seek to remove the cause, and the after results, whatever they may be, will disappear automatically."

- "Healing will pass from the domain of physical methods of treating the physical body to that of spiritual and mental healing, which, by bringing about harmony between the Soul and mind, will eradicate the very basic cause of disease, and then allow such physical means to be used as may be necessary to complete the cure of the body."

- "Our object in life is to follow the dictates of our Higher Self, undeterred by the influence of others, and this can only be achieved if we gently go our own way, but at the same time never interfere with the personality of another or cause the least harm by any method of cruelty or hate."

- "In correct healing nothing must be used which relieves the patient of his own responsibility; but such means only must be adopted which help him to overcome his faults."

- "For those who are sick, peace of mind and harmony with the Soul is the greatest aid to recovery."

- *"We can judge our health by our happiness, and by our happiness we know that we're obeying the dictates of our Souls."*
- *"Sickness and wrong are not to be conquered by direct fighting, but by replacing them by good. Darkness is removed by light, not by greater darkness, hate by love, cruelty by sympathy and pity and disease by health."*
- *"Thus we see that our conquest of disease will mainly depend on the following: firstly, the realization of the Divinity within our nature and our consequent power to overcome all that is wrong; secondly, the knowledge that the basic cause of disease is due to disharmony between the personality and the Soul; thirdly, our willingness and ability to discover the fault which is causing such a conflict; and fourthly, the removal of any such fault by developing the opposing virtue."*

Edward Bach had amazing insights into life and developed his own philosophy about the meaning of life including the topics of health and healing. In so many ways he was well ahead of his times and still is now, in the 21st century. Bach was conscious of his purpose and realized how important this awareness was. When he was diagnosed with terminal cancer in 1917 at the age of 31 he was given only three months to live. Since he kept his focus on his mission in life, which had not been completed, he got well and lived for another 19 years before he passed on in 1936. It was his strong conviction that gave him the strength to persevere and made him understand the significance of hope in healing. Without hope or purpose to live, chances for recovery are greatly reduced.

ADDITIONAL FACTORS TO CONSIDER ON OUR PATH TO WELLNESS

"It must never be forgotten that this (the physical body – author's note) is but the earthly habitation of the Soul, in which we dwell only for a short time in order that we may be able to contact the world for the purpose of gaining experience and knowledge."

—EDWARD BACH

Edward Bach understood the great healing potential of the Bach Flowers which address our emotions and mental states. He recognized these as the most significant factors in the entire spectrum of healing. Even though he believed that we should never pay too much attention to our physical bodies or should allow ourselves to be over-anxious with them, he was aware of the importance of treating our bodies with *"respect and care so that they may be healthy and last the longer to do our work."* (Edward Bach) Despite its relevancy, this fact is rarely mentioned in the context of the Bach Flowers.

Bach recommended the following measures to support our physical body.

- External cleanliness: water for washing ourselves should be cool to tepid and soap should only be used sparingly when necessary.
- Diet referred to as internal cleanliness: vegetarian consisting primarily of fresh fruits, vegetables and nuts; meat should be avoided because, according to Bach, it adds poison in the physical body, stimulates abnormal and excessive appetite and causes cruelty to the animals.

- Adequate fluid intake especially water, and avoiding artificial beverages.
- Sleep, not too much, not too little. He felt that most sleep too much.
- Clothing should be light in weight and allow *"air to reach the body".* (Edward Bach)
- Sunshine and air at any possible occasion.
- Water and sunbathing as *"great donors of health and vitality".* (Edward Bach)

The 21st century brings with it new challenges for our physical bodies that clearly influence our mental, emotional and spiritual well-being. In order to enhance our own healing process and, through that, facilitate the healing of the Earth, we have to find our way back to nature and understand that we are only a small strand in the web of life. We also need to reduce our exposure to electromagnetic background radiation and break the addiction to electronic devices that have caused a breakdown in communication, and despite their benefits, have undesirable side effects.

CHAPTER 5

Discoveries During
Edward Bach's Medical Career

*"Thus teach people, as children of the Creator, the Divine
individuality within them which is able to overcome all
trials and difficulties; help them to steer their ship over the
sea of life, keeping a true course and heeding not others;
and teach them also ever to look ahead, for, however they
may have gone out of their course and whatever storms
and tempests they may have experienced, there is always
ahead for everyone the harbour of peace and security."*

—**EDWARD BACH**

Edward Bach made many significant discoveries during his
medical career. He spent much of his time with research in
his quest for a comprehensive system of healing. At that time he
relied primarily on his intellectual abilities and in order to avoid
distractions from his work he refrained from spending any time
in nature.

DISCOVERIES

- Bach discovered that some intestinal germs, which up to then had been considered relatively unimportant, were closely connected to chronic disease. These bacteria are present in everybody but in increased numbers in sick people.

- Edward Bach found that chronic disease was closely connected to poisoning from certain organisms in the intestinal tract. Once the toxins were removed, the (chronic) complaints disappeared.

- He isolated seven groups of intestinal bacteria and prepared vaccines homeopathically from them. He grouped the bacteria according to their fermentation action on sugars. The vaccines had a purifying effect in the intestines resulting in great improvement. These vaccines were very successful and became known as the seven Bach nosodes. While his fame spread with the nosodes being in high demand, he spent much of his time searching for plants and herbs, hoping to replace the nosodes, but initially had no success.

- Bach realized that all people suffering from the same emotional difficulty needed the same nosode. This confirmed his opinion that dis-ease was not of physical origin but the consolidation of mental attitudes.

- As a result of his heightened intuitive senses and keen observation skills he recognized in 1928 that all of humanity consists of a certain number of definite groups or types.

- Furthermore, Bach discovered that the seven bacterial groups correspond to seven different and definite human personalities. He began treating his patients according to their temperament with results beyond all expectations.

- Members of each group were clearly recognizable by their behaviour, moods or attitudes.

> *"If Tommy gets measles, he may be irritable – Sissy may be quiet and drowsy – Johnny wants to be pitied – little Peter may be all nerves and fearful."*

—EDWARD BACH

Examples: You can observe the different behaviours of people at a beach deciding to go into the water. One person might be nervous and fearful, testing out the water carefully; the next one might be undecided and hesitant, taking time to decide before entering the water; yet another individual might run straight into the water without giving any thought to the temperature of the water or any potential dangers. Each person acts according to their own individuality.

Another example would be in regard to making decisions. Some people have the tendency to base their decisions on avoiding conflict, others allow themselves to be overly influenced by the opinion of others and yet a third group might be over-confident, "knowing" that they are always right.

These examples clearly illustrate how our personality influences our behaviour in different situations. The distinct differences in reactions apply to physical illness as well.

- Each individual belonging to a specific group would not necessarily suffer from the same disease but instead their reaction to disease was similar or the same. Therefore, Bach concluded that a person's reaction to disease was the real key to treatment. The reaction is determined by the personality and provides the criteria for treatment.

- The disease is only a symptom of the cause, and the same cause will manifest itself differently in nearly every individual.

"A small worry passing through the mind will cause a look of strain to appear upon the face, so a continued large worry will have a correspondingly greater effect upon the body; but in both cases as soon as the worrying thought had been removed and the peace and happiness of the mind restored, all the ill effects upon the body will go also."

—NORA WEEKS

These discoveries were the true beginning of finding the new system of healing and became the underlying principles of healing with Bach Flower essences.

CHAPTER 6

Discovery of the Bach Flowers

"To Nature we look confidently for all the needs to keep us alive – air, light, food, drink, and so on, it is not likely that on this great scheme which provides all, the healing of illness and distress should be forgotten."

—EDWARD BACH

Throughout Bach's medical practice and research, it became evident to him that treating the personality rather than the physical disease needed to become the primary focus, the principle of the new system of medicine he sought to develop. He was certain that the source for this new method could be found within the plant world.

Bach had always been a very sensitive person but by 1928 he felt, more than ever before, deeply in tune with his intuition and spirituality. That year he had the inspiration to go to Wales and, following the commands of his Soul, he took a break from his medical practice and the hustle and bustle in London to re-connect with nature. While roaming the tranquil countryside in Wales he came upon two beautiful plants growing by a mountain stream, the pale mauve *Impatiens* and the golden flowered *Mimulus*.

When he returned to London he prepared both of these flowers homeopathically and began treating his patients with them according to their personality and temperament; *Impatiens* for impatience and *Mimulus* for known fears. The results were encouraging. Later in the year he added *Clematis* for the person escaping from the present and displaying indifference and boredom. By the end of 1929 he had given up all other forms of treatment, focusing entirely on the use of these three flower remedies.

All three flowers were later to become part of his new system of healing, known today as the Bach Flower remedies. He eventually parted way with homeopathy and began creating the remedies in a much simpler form, using only the elements of nature. See Chapter 15, *Instructions for Creating Bach Flower Essences,* for further details.

Two years later, at the age of 43, knowing there was more work to be done to complete his mission, he gave up his lucrative medical practice in London completely. Following his intuition, his inner guiding light, he returned to the countrysides of Wales and England, dedicating himself to the search for a gentle, yet effective form of medicine.

Bach invited Nora Weeks, who had worked for him in his Harley Street practice in London, to accompany him on his journey. Nora provided great support to Bach in the following years and it is said that Bach's accomplishments and the continuation of his work after his death would not have been possible without her support and efforts.

From 1930 to 1936 Bach and Nora Weeks spent countless hours traveling along lakes, rivers, fields and in the mountains, searching among nature for the plants he knew would provide true healing to humankind. He prepared and tested a large number of plants, some say thousands, before he found the ones he was looking for.

His intuition and senses became increasingly sensitive and heightened which enabled him to communicate with nature in a very clear and intimate way. He began to see, hear and feel things that he had not been conscious of before. Bach was drawn to work with the flowers of plants because he instinctively knew that the flowers themselves hold within them all the potential energy and vitality of a plant. The flower is like the signature of the plant, containing the personality and spirit within its vibrational frequencies which creates its potential for healing.

Bach realized that he was able to communicate with the spirit of the plants, feeling their vibrations by placing the flower, or parts of the plant, in his hand or on his tongue. By doing so he could feel in his body the different effects of the properties of the flower such as strength, vitality or pain. He then discovered that the dew drops resting on the flowers carried the same properties as the actual plant material and that dew drops exposed to the sun were stronger in their effect than the ones collected from the shade. This eventually led him to develop his method of preparation of the flower essences using the elements of nature.

> *"It was the method of simplicity he had longed for– the simplicity of mighty things, for fire, earth, air and water–the four elements–were involved and working together to produce healing remedies of great power."*
>
> **—NORA WEEKS**

By 1932 Bach had discovered the first 12 Bach Flowers and he wrote his book *The Twelve Healers* which corresponded to the 12 main groups or types of individuals that he had isolated.

From 1932 to 1934 he found seven more flowers to be part
of his new medicine and he also developed the *Rescue Remedy*,
a combination of five Bach Flower essences, for use in emergencies and times of great distress. At that time he believed his work
to be complete but later realized that more flowers were required
in order to address the great variations of personalities, emotions
and mental states.

From 1934 to 1936 he found the remaining 19 remedies from
flowers, and buds and flowers from trees and bushes. On his quest
for the missing flowers Edward Bach suffered for each one of them
the emotional state, including distressing physical challenges,
until he found the one single plant or flower required to overcome
the situation. At times he was so sick that people around him were
surprised that he was able to recover. Fulfilling his purpose in life
was driven by such an intensity that it was hard to understand for
most and therefore he often went through life alone.

In the beginning Bach had thought that each flower focused
primarily either on acute, chronic or more spiritual aspects but
dismissed this idea as time went on.

While discovering the flowers, Bach continued to observe
people, studying their moods and reactions. This confirmed
his original observations that humanity is divided into definite
personality types. He continued to treat patients accordingly and
the results convinced him that he had finally found the method of
healing that he had been looking for.

In the summer of 1936 he wrote the final edition of *The Twelve
Healers and Other Remedies* reflecting the completion of his work.
In order to avoid potential confusion in the future he burnt all his
previous writings in a bonfire.

Throughout the period of discovering and preparing the new

plant medicines Bach remained true to his ideals and treated patients free of charge.

BACH FLOWERS ACCORDING TO TIME OF DISCOVERY

1930 – 1932

Agrimony	– Cheerful facade
Centaury	– Subservience
Cerato	– Self-doubt
Chicory	– Possessiveness, selfishness
*Clematis	– Mental escapism
Gentian	– Despondency
*Impatiens	– Irritation
*Mimulus	– Fear and shyness
Rock Rose	– Terror
Scleranthus	– Indecision
Vervain	– Over-enthusisam
Water Violet	– Pride

* The original discovery of these three flowers was in 1928; as of 1930 Bach began preparing the remedies with the sun and boiling method he had developed rather than homeopathically and therefore the discovery date is usually listed as 1930.

1932 – 1934

Gorse	– Hopelessness
Heather	– Loneliness, self-centeredness
Oak	– Struggling, never giving up
Olive	– Exhaustion
Rock Water	– Lack of flexibility

Vine   – Desire to influence others
Wild Oat   – Uncertainty, lack of direction

1935–1936

Aspen   – Undefined fear
Beech   – Intolerance
Cherry Plum   – Irrational thoughts, hysteria
Chestnut Bud   – Repetition of mistakes
Crab Apple   – Self-disgust
Elm   – Burden of responsibility
Holly   – Hatred, jealousy, suspicion
Honeysuckle   – Homesickness, nostalgia, living in the past
Hornbeam   – Procrastination
Larch   – Lack of confidence
Mustard   – Unexplained depression
Pine   – Guilt
Red Chestnut   – Anxiety for others
Star of Bethlehem – Shock and sorrow
Sweet Chestnut   – Despair
Walnut   – Adjustment
White Chestnut   – Worry
Wild Rose   – Apathetic resignation
Willow   – Resentment

CHAPTER 7

The Seven Categories

"Nothing in nature can hurt us when we are happy and in harmony, on the contrary all nature is there for our use and our enjoyment."

—EDWARD BACH

As a result of Edward Bach's observations he concluded that all of humanity consists of only seven different, primary types of personalities with each group having sub-categories. He applied this information to the Bach Flowers by assigning each flower to one of the seven groups, each of them referring to a major emotion or mental state.

The seven categories (personality types) are: Fear, uncertainty, insufficient interest in present circumstances, loneliness, over-sensitivity to influences and ideas from others, despondency and despair, over-care for welfare of others.

The usefulness of this form of classification has been questioned by many and abandoned by some because over time additional information has been revealed by the flowers which can make it difficult to assign them to Bach's original groupings. In this respect classifying the flowers according to the original system may create limitations.

If one regards the classification as a rigid system this view is true. However, Bach's categories can also be seen as a free flowing system without "definite boundaries" meaning that individual Bach Flowers can belong to different groups. Depending on where a person is in their life, the momentary situation, support needed and learning required, flower essences will bring forth different aspects. The descriptions of the Bach Flowers can only serve as a guide because the flower essences have so much more to offer than can be expressed verbally or comprehended by our limited human mind. Their innate intelligence will bring forth the qualities that best harmonize with the person looking for support and guidance, yet their main focus remains as initially designated by Edward Bach. Looking at the seven groups in this context, the original division is still of great value.

For any person wanting to work with the Bach Flowers the seven groups provide a great self-help tool for choosing an appropriate remedy. For example, a person dealing with fears may check the flowers of that category and find out which one would be the most relevant. Keep in mind that this method of choosing flower essences, even though very beneficial, has some limitations. When our choices are based on our conscious mind we do not always get to the real cause or source of our challenges because our mind is powerful and can distort reality for a variety of reasons.

Bach's original classification can be correlated to the main chakras of the body. The word chakra originates from Sanskrit meaning "wheel". These wheels are defined as energy centers within and outside of the body connecting us to outside sources of energy. They transfer information from the universe and regulate physical, mental, emotional and spiritual processes. Each chakra has its own vibrational frequency that resonates to a very specific colour.

As the Earth is evolving into higher vibrational frequencies so is the chakra system changing with it. These new developments are not well known or accepted yet but over time this will change.

Bach defined the seven categories by their limiting emotion and I have added the desirable, positive attribute, the one that the flower essence can help a person achieve. Following is a list of the seven groups including the flowers belonging to each.

Note that I have listed the positive attribute before Bach's original classification (in italics) not out of disrespect for Bach's work but because it is important to bring forward the positive aspects to further illuminate Bach's idea about healing. It is the positive virtue that we want to uphold: "*... to open up those channels to admit more of the light of the Soul, that the patient may be flooded with healing virtue.*" (Edward Bach)

1. **Sense of security – *Fear***
   Flowers: *Aspen, Cherry Plum, Mimulus, Red Chestnut, Rock Rose*

2. **Sense of certainty and self-worth as a result of trust in inner knowing – *To those who suffer uncertainty***
   Flowers: *Cerato, Gentian, Gorse, Hornbeam, Scleranthus, Wild Oat*

3. **Staying focused in the present in all that you know – *Insufficient interest in present circumstances***
   Flowers: *Chestnut Bud, Clematis, Honeysuckle, Mustard, Olive, White Chestnut, Wild Rose*

4. **Nurture and support sense of trust and belonging – *Loneliness***
   Flowers: *Heather, Impatiens, Water Violet*

5. **Strength to stay focused and true to one's own ideals –** *Over-sensitivity to influences and ideas from others*
Flowers: *Agrimony, Centaury, Holly, Walnut*

6. **Encouragement and contentment with heightened capacity for spiritual knowledge –** *Despondency and despair*
Flowers: *Crab Apple, Elm, Larch, Oak, Pine, Star of Bethlehem, Sweet Chestnut, Willow*

7. **Living in synchronized balance and understanding of the highest (heart woven) truth –** *Over-care for welfare of others*
Flowers: *Beech, Chicory, Rock Water, Vervain, Vine*

RESCUE REMEDY

Clarity and strength for inner peace – *Stress and trauma*
Flower Combination as one remedy: *Clematis, Rock Rose, Cherry Plum, Impatiens, Star of Bethlehem*

CHAPTER 8

Rescue Remedy

"Simple, natural and gentle acting, the Bach Flower Remedies provide a wonderful tool to help our inherent ability to restore balance and harmony within ourselves."

—EDWARD BACH

Rescue Remedy is a combination of five Bach Flower essences. Bach developed this combination as a first-aid remedy to be used in case of emergencies or stressful situations that cause feelings such as fear, shock, panic, anxiety and loss of consciousness. Regardless of the magnitude of the circumstances, small or large, *Rescue Remedy* with its calming and comforting effect can lend a helping hand like a best friend whenever we have lost our balance. The flower essences help to restore balance quickly by assisting one to stay present and giving the strength and courage to adequately deal with the situation.

The *Rescue Remedy* minimizes the possibility of a traumatic event being imprinted long-term into a person's cellular memory.

This is of great benefit because too often trauma can have life long consequences, causing limiting emotions and mental states which create restrictions to future growth and development, holding us back from being all we could be.

For example, a child getting bit by a dog may easily develop a fear of dogs for the rest of her life. Taking the *Rescue Remedy* right away or shortly after the event, the high vibrational frequencies of the flower essences will instantly fill the child's being with its positive, healing virtues, making it less likely for the event to be locked into cellular memory. The child will be able to process the traumatic event as an isolated experience rather than store it as fear that "all dogs are dangerous".

The *Rescue Remedy* includes:

- *Cherry Plum:* For fear of losing control of one's thoughts and actions
- *Star of Bethlehem:* For trauma and shock
- *Impatiens:* For impatience
- *Rock Rose:* For extreme fear, panic or terror
- *Clematis:* For staying present in the moment

EXAMPLES OF THE APPLICATION OF RESCUE REMEDY – FOR HUMANS, ANIMALS AND PLANTS

- During and right after any stressful, traumatic experiences, accidents and injuries
- Exams and interviews
- Doctor and dentist visit
- Surgery and other medical procedures – blood work, x-rays, MRIs
- Travel – airplane travel, challenging situations, home sickness, taking pets to a vet

- Family/home life – unsettled children, rebellious teen-agers, relationship crisis
- Sickness – self and others; accompanying a friend or family member during severe illness or transition
- Feeling "shaken up" by disturbing news or a film
- Dog bites or bites from other animals
- Anticipation of a stressful situation
- Anything that causes loss of mental balance
- Whenever you have the need for support
- Animals – fear of thunder, separation anxiety, introduction of another animal into the household, travel
- Plants – transplanting, illness, neglect

Once the crisis is over the use of the *Rescue Remedy* should be discontinued and if necessary, be replaced with an individualized Bach Flower essence.

RESCUE REMEDY AND A CLINICAL TRIAL

According to the Bach Centre in England researchers at the University of Miami School of Nursing conducted a double-blind clinical trial with the *Rescue Remedy* for the use in anxiety. The study involved 111 individuals, aged 18 to 49. It included a standardized test for the evaluation of anxiety and was administered before and after the intake of *Rescue Remedy*.

The results showed that the *Rescue Remedy* was *"an effective over-the-counter stress reliever with a comparable effect to traditional pharmaceutical drugs yet without any of the known adverse side effects, including addiction."* (Medical News Today, July 2, 2007)

Statistics suggest that 40 million Americans are diagnosed by physicians with anxiety. Ronald Stram, MD, regularly prescribes *Rescue Remedy* to his anxious and stressed patients.

"Stress compromises your ability to fight off disease and infection. It can even rewire the brain, making you more vulnerable to everyday pressures and problems." (Ronald Stram, MD, Medical News Today, July 2, 2007). Taking these facts into account, the *Rescue Remedy* can be considered as first line of defense in stressful situations including anxiety as well as a preventative measure in reducing the risk of dis-ease.

CHAPTER 9

Detailed Description of
the Bach Flowers and Working Guide

*"Has it ever occurred to you that God gave you an
individuality? Yet he certainly did. He gave you a personality
of your very own, a treasure to be kept to your very own self.
He gave you a life to lead that you and only you should lead.
He gave you work to do that you and only you can do. He
placed you in this world, a Divine being, a child of himself
– to learn how to become perfect, to gain all knowledge
possible, to grow gentle and kind, and to help others."*

—EDWARD BACH

In this chapter you will find detailed descriptions about each of
the 38 Bach Flowers plus the *Rescue Remedy*. You can use this
part of the book as a working tool, a self-help guide to support
you on your healing journey whether you are looking for answers
for a short term situation or need assistance and direction in long
term challenges. If you simply want to deepen your knowledge

about the Bach Flowers this chapter provides you with a wealth of information.

The chapter has been organized according to the seven categories as originally developed by Edward Bach. In order to make it easier to find a specific flower you might be looking for, an alphabetical index has been included following this introduction.

The material presented about each Bach Flower includes the following:

- **Image** – Photograph or art of the respective Bach Flower. The artwork is taken from *Bach Flowers Unfolding*.
- **Message** – Channeled through communication with plant spirit which can be used as an affirmation.
- **Focus** – The major aspects (emotions, mental states) the Bach Flower addresses.
- **Category** – The category as assigned by Edward Bach including his description along with the transformed state. Note that I have listed the positive attribute before Bach's original classification (in italics) not out of disrespect for Bach's work but because it is important to bring forward the positive aspects to further illuminate Bach's idea about healing.
- **Chakras** – The numbers relating to the chakras the Bach Flower primarily influences.
- **Colours** – The colour frequencies brought forth by the flower (unrelated to the chakras)
- **Number** – For those who work with the vibrational frequencies of numbers each flower resonates to a specific number.
- **Detailed descriptions** – Challenges we are experiencing and the possibilities of the transformed states. The issue(s)

addressed may relate to a current event, a short term situation or a long-term, underlying theme of your life.

NOTE: The descriptions focus on the key aspects to which each Bach Flower relates. However, the essences bring forth many more energies than can be included here but the ones relevant for a person at a given time will be the ones conveyed by the flowers.

Please note that the essence of Edward Bach's original work has been carefully preserved. Many decades have passed since Bach developed this remarkable method of healing but times are changing and the increase in the vibrational frequencies of the planet affects not only humankind but all life forms. The information and healing possibilities brought forth by the Bach Flowers are adjusting to these changes although the core values remain the same.

Bach himself talked about the vibrations of the Bach Flowers and one can safely assume that he would recognize how the current evolutionary changes on this planet are affecting the Bach Flowers as well. The information has been given to me through intuitive communication with the spirit of the Bach Flowers and through the spiritual guidance of Edward Bach himself.

HOW TO WORK WITH THIS CHAPTER

*"We should strive to be so gentle, so quiet, so patiently
helpful that we move among our fellow men more as a
breath of air or a ray of sunshine; ever ready to help them
when they ask: but never forcing them to our own views."*

—EDWARD BACH

As outlined in Chapter 11, *Practical Information – Methods and
Practical Guidelines for Selecting Bach Flowers*, when you are not
certain about which Bach Flower(s) might be needed, narrowing
the choice down by first selecting the appropriate category can
be beneficial. Once you have decided on the category, reading
the descriptions relating to each flower will help you find the
one(s) you want to bring into your life.

Another option is to look at the images and work with the one(s)
you feel most attracted to. You can do the same by reading the text.

Some people may simply open the book and work with that
specific flower. Once you have made your choice, be creative and
trust your intuition on how to best incorporate the information
into your daily life. Following are some suggestions.

- Look at the image and/or read the text and receive the
  information with an open heart and mind. Do this
  several times daily or at least morning and/or night.
- Work with the message, use it as an affirmation.
- Incorporate the colours suggested into your life through
  clothing, colour bath, food etc.
- If you have the *Bach Flowers Unfolding* cards, choose
  the ones you wish to work with and keep them with you
  or put them on the fridge or any other place you pass
  frequently throughout the day.

- Get a treatment bottle and work with the actual remedies.
- Journal your experiences – before and after. Keeping a journal can be a great companion. Writing our experiences allows for the movement of energy providing healing. Be observant of any changes – physical, mental, emotional and spiritual. Journaling makes us more conscious of any changes; many times we are not aware of our progress, especially the more subtle changes because we so readily adjust to small improvements and forget what life was like before.
- For more ideas see Chapter 13, *How to Get to Know the Bach Flowers.*

ALPHABETICAL INDEX OF BACH FLOWERS

CATEGORY 1:

- Sense of Security – *Fear*
- <u>Flowers:</u> *Aspen, Cherry Plum, Mimulus, Red Chestnut, Rock Rose*

ASPEN

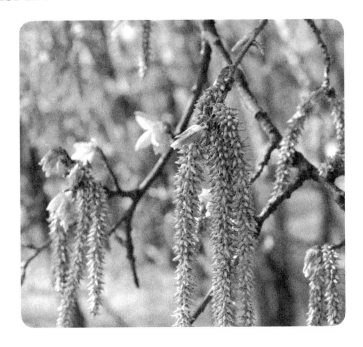

MESSAGE: I, Aspen, am a tree of high frequency. I will shine a bright light, brilliant pearl, bringing transparency and clarity, comfort and ease, enlightening every part of your being.

FOCUS: Comfort – Clarity – Trust – Clairvoyance – Stillness

CATEGORY: Sense of security – *Fear*

CHAKRAS: 1, 2, 5

COLOURS: Gold – Green – Turquoise

NUMBER: 16

Our intuition is like a channel of communication with the invisible worlds. It allows us to tune into information given by our Soul, the inner child, and energies all around us in the universe. You are gifted with an exceptional intuitive/clairvoyant sense; however you are not conscious of your potentially strong connection to the universe. You have the tendency to doubt your intuition. Some events may create a sense of uneasiness as well as fears and uncertainties within you. You do not seem to be able to explain these sensations that may haunt you day and night, and might wonder where they are coming from. You may feel anxious, restless, vulnerable and "uncomfortable in your own skin".

Aspen is a tree of high frequencies that vibrates harmoniously with your gentle and sensitive nature, bringing clarity to your spirit connection and the energies of the invisible worlds that move freely through and around you. Aspen encourages you to develop your gift of sensitivity so that you may become all that you are. As love and light from Aspen fill your being, you will hear and understand spirit clearly, learning to trust your intuition and spiritual knowing. Fears will dissolve and be replaced with stillness. Your sensitivity, gentleness and softness will become your strength because you know that you are safe and protected at all times. You will touch many peoples' lives, bringing clarity in a subtle and gentle way. You are a being of high frequency, radiating gently, spreading love, light and healing wherever you go.

CHERRY PLUM

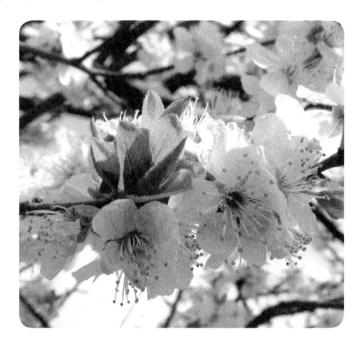

MESSAGE:	Breathe my essence in deeply. I, Cherry Plum, assist you in restoring harmony and calmness in your life by transforming fears into trust, synchronized balance and light.
FOCUS:	Harmonics – Opening channels – Sense of connecting above to below – Tranquility of mind
CATEGORY:	Sense of security – *Fear*
CHAKRAS:	1, 4
COLOURS:	Green – Gold – Pearl
NUMBER:	20

You are very connected to your spirit and are an open channel for the universal love energy; however you are not fully aware of your gift. This lack of awareness creates feelings and sensations within you that seem beyond your control. Fears of "losing your mind" that could result in unreasonable thoughts and actions are haunting you. Your imagination may become irrationally fearful, creating deeper fear-based emotions of unknown origin. As a result, you are experiencing moments of discomfort, internal tension and fear that may intensify to panic.

Cherry Plum has incredible strength and is willing to share this freely with you. It creates an instant grounding effect, giving you a sense of security and tranquility of mind. Cherry Plum fills all aspects of your being with radiant light, creating harmonious vibrations and an understanding of why you are feeling, thinking and acting the way you are. Fears will diminish and transform into pure light creating peace, balance and trust. Being conscious of your strong, innate spirit connection will keep your channels to spirit and the universal love energy clear and free flowing. It will give you strength and allow you to receive and give love freely, living a life in harmony and synchronized balance.

MIMULUS

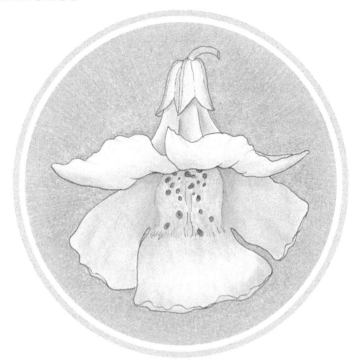

MESSAGE:	Trust in me and I will guide you to gently embrace your fears, releasing them to the universe, setting you free and allowing you the freedom to be all who you are meant to be.
FOCUS:	Trust – Embracing fears – Courage
CATEGORY:	Sense of security – *Fear*
CHAKRAS:	1, 4, 5
COLOURS:	Pink – Pearl – Gold – Yellow
NUMBER:	26

Fear, a feeling well known to all of us, can be a challenging stumbling block as we move forward on our journey through life. Fear causes restriction and congestion, interfering with our connection to spirit and the free flow of the life force. You are harboring some worldly fears such as fear of the dark, fear of illness, fear of spiders or other animals, fear of being alone, being loved or expressing love. These fears are locked into your cellular memory and are holding you back from being all you truly are in your entire beauty.

Mimulus encourages you to embrace your fears. Its compassionate vibrational frequencies will nurture and support you, bringing light to your fears, making it easier to let go. You will find the courage, strength and trust to release what is holding you back from being all who you are. As your fears gently fade away, your trust in your connection to your true spiritual essence will blossom and shine. With the help of Mimulus you will spread your wings, soaring to new heights, discovering and unfolding your beautiful, true, loving and caring self. You will radiate a golden light on this Earth like the sun in the sky.

RED CHESTNUT

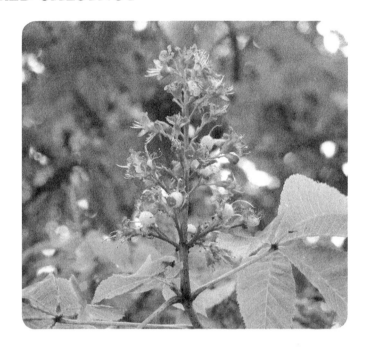

MESSAGE: I, Red Chestnut, encourage balance and
                harmony in your life by radiating clarity and
                understanding, transforming imbalances into
                love and light energy.

FOCUS: Trust – Balance – Serenity

CATEGORY: Sense of security – *Fear*

CHAKRAS: 1, 2, 7

COLOURS: White – Indigo – Blue – Pink

NUMBER: 6

Communicating, sharing and caring for each other are integral parts of our everyday life. You have the natural ability to care for your family and friends; their well-being is of great importance and concern to you. However, in your situation caring for others easily turns into being worried and anxious about them. You seem to be more concerned with their needs than your own. Realize that your well-meant actions and worrying thoughts may interfere with the free will of the people you care about, creating disharmony, fear, anxiety, insecurities and lack of trust on deep levels of the subconscious. Your worrying will make it more challenging for them to live life in harmony with their own true Soul essence and therefore unfold to their full potential.

Red Chestnut guides you gently and with love to trust in Divine guidance so that your fear for others will transform into tranquility, peace and harmony. You will begin to shine like a beautiful light radiating calm and confidence. You will be able to give support and comfort to the ones near to you without influencing their lives in an undesirable way. Red Chestnut also brings clarity to your own Soul essence, helping you to recognize and understand your own needs and desires as they deserve equal attention. Listen with your heart to Red Chestnut, follow its guidance and all will be well.

ROCK ROSE

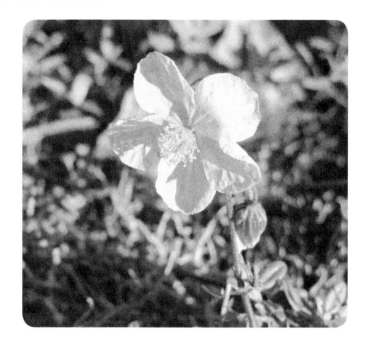

MESSAGE: Trust and I will illuminate your being with golden light, giving you the courage and power to heal.

FOCUS: Calmness – Peace – Grounding – Healing

CATEGORY: Sense of security – *Fear*

CHAKRAS: 1, 2, 3, 8 (thymus)

COLOURS: Gold – Yellow – Green – Violet

NUMBER: 24

Life is filled with a great variety of experiences some of which may be truly disturbing, causing trauma and overpowering feelings of fear, anxiety and possibly terror. We, and/or the people around us, may feel hopeless and lost, finding it hard to trust that life will improve again. These emotions create energy blockages in all aspects of our being, interfering with the free flow of the life force and therefore with the healing process. You are currently living through such a crisis, feeling numb and almost paralyzed with intense, deep-seated fear. Your connection to spirit is broken, making it difficult to have faith and trust in the process of life and slowing your possibilities for healing and moving forward.

Rock Rose imparts great strength and courage, renewing your trust and power to heal. Your fears will fade away, allowing your connection to your Soul essence to return with clarity. Rock Rose will ground you and bring light to the events that are causing you the disruptive feelings of fear and terror. Energy blockages will dissipate, encouraging you to once again fill your being with the rejuvenating breath of life. Rock Rose shares love and light freely with you, filling your essence with peace and harmony and the power to heal. Joy and happiness will return, allowing you to continue to create balance and security through giving light to all life within and around you.

REFLECTIONS

CATEGORY 2:

- Sense of Certainty and Self-Worth as a Result of Trust in Inner Knowing - *To Those Who Suffer Uncertainty*
- <u>Flowers:</u> **Cerato, Gentian, Gorse, Hornbeam, Scleranthus, Wild Oat**

CERATO

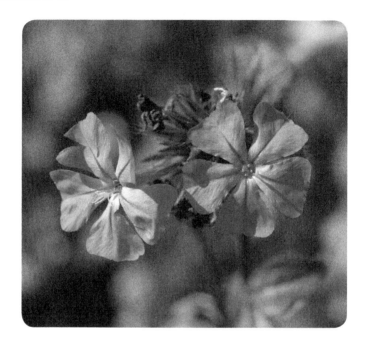

MESSAGE: I, Cerato, guide you so that you may walk with confidence on this Earth, radiating all you know and dwelling in the energies of frequencies of light.

FOCUS: Trust – Strength – Inner guidance

CATEGORY: Sense of certainty and self-worth as a result of trust in inner knowing – *To those who suffer uncertainty*

CHAKRAS: 2, 3

COLOURS: Blue – Violet – White

NUMBER: 2

We may have the strong desire to live with confidence and universal guidance but may experience uncertainty in both. At this moment you are challenged with a lack of confidence and trust in your intuition making it difficult for you to make your own decisions and to walk through life with clarity and clear focus. You have the tendency to depend on the advice of others, giving away your own power and at times allowing yourself to be led astray. This lack of confidence in your own abilities is interfering with your inner knowing and trust in your otherwise strong, innate intuitive senses.

Cerato strengthens your connection to spirit. With gentleness and love, the essence will guide you to listen with your heart, increasing your awareness and consciousness. You will enjoy a heightened sense of your intuitive abilities and learn to trust and follow them. With renewed confidence in your own strength and knowing, you will once again be able to make your own decisions easily and live your life in accordance with your true Soul essence. Cerato fills you with abundant, radiant light giving you joy, strength, peace and harmony, allowing your life to flow with ease.

GENTIAN

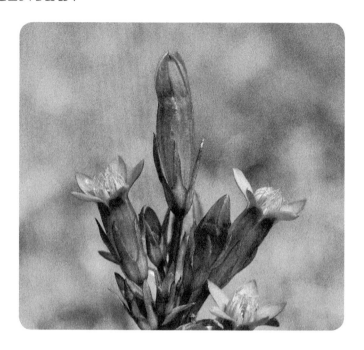

MESSAGE: I, Gentian, am of high vibrational frequency.
Like gentle music from the ultimate source,
I am filling your being with love and light,
encouraging you to move forward with ease.

FOCUS: Trust in universal guidance – Gentleness –
Strength – Faith

CATEGORY: Sense of certainty and self-worth as a result
of trust in inner knowing – *To those who
suffer uncertainty*

CHAKRAS: 1, 7

COLOURS: Green – Violet – Lime green – Gold – White

NUMBER: 22

Life is forever evolving. Some moments we experience joy and are able to see the beauty in all there is. At other times life presents itself with challenges, small and large, which provide many opportunities for learning and personal growth. You easily feel overwhelmed by challenges and set-backs. When things go "wrong" you experience doubt, feel disheartened and alone in this world. You question your connection to spirit and at times it feels like you have lost your trust in universal guidance and the process of life, not expecting to succeed in accomplishing your goals.

Gentian vibrates with incredible gentleness and kindness; forever reminding us of our constant connection to the Higher Spirit and Mother Earth. Gentian increases your awareness of the ever-presence of the universal love energy, creating synchronized balance, strengthening your trust and belief that you are always being taken care of regardless of the circumstances you encounter in your life. Gentian will open your channels that connect you to the universe, encouraging the free flow of universal love and life force. You will feel and experience this love in a most profound way, creating new levels of trust and faith. With deepened trust in universal guidance you will be able to embrace life with more confidence and new strength. Small challenges will no longer create doubt and leave you disheartened because you truly know that, in the end, everything will work out. Life will begin to flow with ease.

GORSE

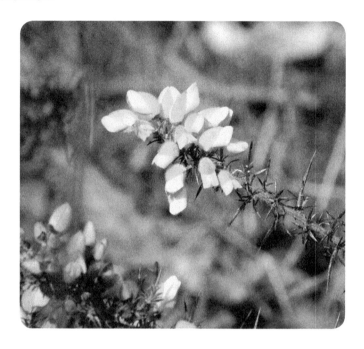

MESSAGE: Open your heart to my vibrations of synchronized balance so that this energy may flow freely
through you, transforming darkness into light,
filling your being with hope and healing.

FOCUS: Opening of own space – Hope – Healing –
Joy – Grounding

CATEGORY: Sense of certainty and self-worth as a result
of trust in inner knowing – *To those who
suffer uncertainty*

CHAKRAS: 1, 4, 7

COLOURS: Yellow – Green – White

NUMBER: 34

We have all experienced moments of desperation and hope-lessness. However, you have lost the spark for life and feel that there is no hope for improvement. Your misery may be physical, mental, emotional and/or spiritual. You have not been able to find long lasting relief to help you out of this space of darkness. Your heart feels heavy; you have lost your vitality and maybe even the desire to continue with life. Your faith has been shattered and you are feeling betrayed by life and certain that there is little hope for relief.

Gorse fills your being with the loving and life giving energy of the sun, supporting you with hope and courage so that you may live again with joy and certainty. You will receive healing from the vibrational frequencies of Gorse. They will open your space and lift your spirits, allowing you to move through these dark moments more easily. Gorse is here for you, supporting you while you find your connection to spirit, your inner knowing and trust, allowing you to live your life with clear direction and focus. Joy and vitality will return. You will blossom like a beautiful flower, shine like the sun and unfold and live according to your true Soul essence.

HORNBEAM

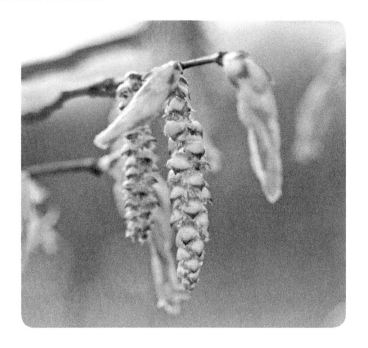

MESSAGE:	I, Hornbeam, bring joy and certainty to your life so that all that you have chosen to accomplish will flow with ease in a positive light.
FOCUS:	Achievement – Ease – Confidence – Joy
CATEGORY:	Sense of certainty and self-worth as a result of trust in inner knowing – *To those who suffer uncertainty*
CHAKRAS:	1, 5, 6
COLOURS:	White – Silver – Yellow – Pearl
NUMBER:	37

There are moments in life when we feel drained of our vitality, left feeling almost lifeless. Your life is presently overshadowed by a heavy cloud, causing lack of joy and motivation. Even though deep down within, you sense and know that joy and vitality will return, it feels like you have temporarily lost the ability to see and connect to your inner glorious light. You feel like an empty vessel, lacking confidence, interest and energy to continue to speak your truth in support of the Earth.

The vibrations of Hornbeam are creating a song of happiness, light and laughter within you, encouraging you to once again focus on the joy and beauty of life. Hornbeam's song re-opens your channels of communication with the universe, nourishing your Soul so that you will once again find the spark of life that lightens your being. The breath of life that allows energy to flow naturally and effortlessly will return. Vitality and higher vibrational frequencies will be restored, allowing you to create your life with certainty and ease.

SCLERANTHUS

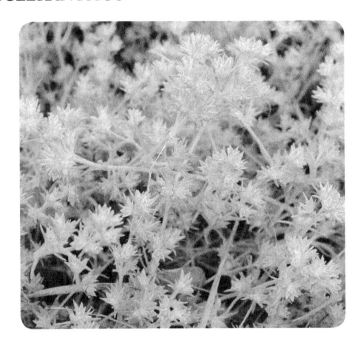

MESSAGE: I, Scleranthus, will simplify your life by giving
you clear direction, making it easy for you to
walk with great confidence on this Earth.

FOCUS: Clarity – Peace – Decisiveness

CATEGORY: Sense of certainty and self-worth as a result
of trust in inner knowing – *To those who
suffer uncertainty*

CHAKRAS: 2, 4, 5

COLOURS: Blue – Turquoise – White

NUMBER: 39

Decision making is an integral part of everyday life; some decisions are minor whereas others have far reaching consequences. When our connection to spirit and the universal love energy is flowing freely, decisions come easily and effortlessly. You have great difficulty at times making decisions. It feels like a process that requires great effort and energy causing you inner turmoil and even torment. Once you have made a decision, you often feel uneasy about it and continue to question yourself. Since you do not wish others to know about your challenges you frequently keep the agony and uncertainty to yourself.

Scleranthus will support you in your everyday life by strengthening your spiritual connection. It will bring clarity, peace and decisiveness, allowing you to make decisions more easily. You will learn to listen with your feelings, trust your intuition and experience a new sense of self-worth. Feelings of uncertainty will transform into confidence, bringing peace and harmony and guiding you to live your life with ease.

WILD OAT

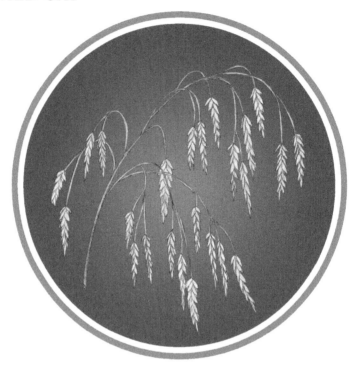

MESSAGE: Feel my energy like the touch of a gentle
                breeze, stroking you with the essence of light,
                illuminating your being, bringing clarity and
                guidance to your Soul.

FOCUS: Playfulness – Clarity – Destiny – Grounding
                – Self realization

CATEGORY: Sense of certainty and self-worth as a result
                of trust in inner knowing – *To those who
                suffer uncertainty*

CHAKRAS: 1, 3, 7

COLOURS: White – Green – Peach – Violet

NUMBER: 7

We enter into our physical existence on this Earth with specific gifts, our Soul's purpose as well as clear guidance and direction. Over time we may lose sight of our connection to our true Soul essence, making it challenging to unfold to our full potential. Yet our physical, mental, emotional and spiritual well-being depends on this process. You have a strong, innate desire to follow your Soul's guidance and fulfill your life's destiny. You wish to accomplish something of importance. However, you are uncertain of what exactly your calling in life is. You are consciously searching but lack clear direction and focus. You are being pulled in many different directions leaving you with feelings of confusion and dissatisfaction.

Wild Oat brings clarity to you, helping you to recognize your destiny. You will become a true conductor of spiritual knowledge, clearly recognizing your Soul essence, allowing you to live your life with focus and direction. Wild Oat assists you in grounding to Mother Earth. You will feel a strong connection and a steady flow of energy between "Heaven and Earth", assisting you in being all that you desire to be and achieving all that you set out to accomplish. Moments of dissatisfaction and confusion will gently melt away and you will be able to move through life with ease.

REFLECTIONS

CATEGORY 3:

- Staying Focused in the Present in All that You Know - *Insufficient Interest in Present Circumstances*
- <u>Flowers:</u> **Chestnut Bud, Clematis, Honeysuckle, Mustard, Olive, White Chestnut, Wild Rose**

CHESTNUT BUD

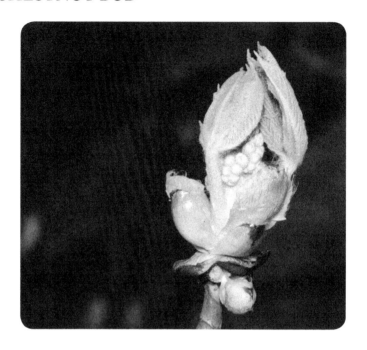

MESSAGE: I, Chestnut Bud, bring consciousness to
every moment of your life and guide you to
understand the purpose of your experiences that
create possibilities for growth and new goals.

FOCUS: Increased awareness – Learning from
experiences – Focus

CATEGORY: Staying focused in the present in all
that you know – *Insufficient interest in
present circumstances*

CHAKRAS: 1, 3

COLOURS: Brown – Silver – Lime green

NUMBER: 32

Life presents itself with many opportunities for learning and personal growth on all levels of our being – physical, mental, emotional and spiritual. Seeing these so called challenges as a gift and embracing them with an open heart ensures continuous movement and evolution in one's life. Due to lack of awareness you tend to only learn slowly from your experiences. Therefore, your life is lacking an easy flow forward and presents itself like a cycle of reoccurring events. It feels like you are trapped in the budding stage, not realizing the benefits of living consciously, and that you do have the tools and power within you to change and move forward.

Chestnut Bud helps you to live with increased awareness and focus so that you may transform from the budding stage into the most beautiful being, radiating courage and strength. You will become conscious of your experiences and embrace situations with new clarity and understanding, allowing you to grow and live in accordance with your Soul essence. Life will flow with ease and like a brilliant flower you will blossom and shine.

CLEMATIS

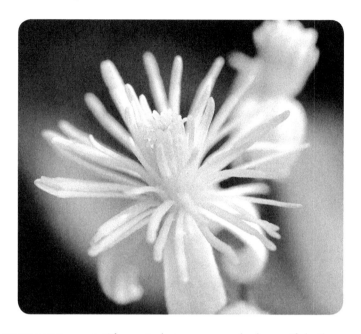

MESSAGE: I, Clematis, bring to you the beautiful vibrations of our Mother Earth guiding you in
shifting your focus from dreaming of the "moon
and the stars" to who you are and to your direction in life. Be conscious of the moment and
you will live your dreams.

FOCUS: Shifting focus to present – Grounding –
Connecting to core – Creativity

CATEGORY: Staying focused in the present in all
that you know – *Insufficient interest in
present circumstances*

CHAKRAS: 2, 3, 6

COLOURS: Green – Violet – Silver – Indigo

NUMBER: 12

Dreams have assisted mankind in amazing ways and will always continue to do so. Dreaming can take on many different forms and dreaming of the future can be useful as long as we do not lose sight of the present. Currently you are longing for a brighter, more joyful future, paying little attention to your present circumstances. This lack of consciousness leaves you feeling disconnected, scattered and without focus and direction. Living in the future causes you to lose sight of opportunities which would allow you to unfold your many gifts and create a harmonious, joyful present.

Clematis guides you in shifting your focus from dreaming of the future and happier times to the present, allowing you to live your life more consciously in the moment with clarity and direction. Without losing sight of what lies ahead, you will discover your gifts and opportunities to live in accordance with your true Soul essence. Clematis gives you a strong sense of balance between living in the present and envisioning your future. In a joyful way you will be able to live your dreams in the here and now.

HONEYSUCKLE

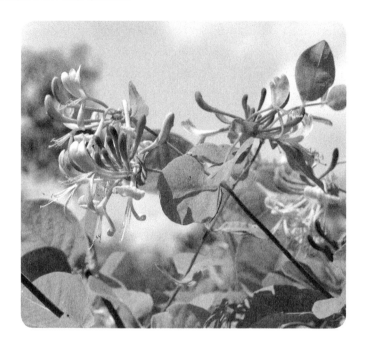

MESSAGE: I, Honeysuckle support your true Soul essence by releasing the past. Sunshine will fill your heart, guiding you to embrace the present.

FOCUS: Cleansing cellular memory – Perception – Integrating all times in the present

CATEGORY: Staying focused in the present in all that you know – *Insufficient interest in present circumstances*

CHAKRAS: 1, 4

COLOURS: Yellow – Gold – Blue

NUMBER: 36

We are like a beautiful tree. The root system represents our life's experiences, nurturing our personal growth and the tree itself mirrors who we are and may become. In order to be able to unfold to our full potential we need to stay conscious in the present moment. You tend to dwell on memories from the past, possibly not even expecting future happiness. Opportunities to move forward pass by you unnoticed, slowing or halting your personal growth. Your lack of interest in present day circumstances hinders you in seeing the beauty and wonder that every moment holds.

Honeysuckle teaches you how to acknowledge the importance of your past without holding on to it. It will assist and encourage you to gently integrate all times – past, past lives, present and future – into the present. It will do so by supporting you in cleansing your cellular memory, thereby creating a shift in your perception of your present life's circumstances. Shifting your focus to the here and now will allow you to see the magnificent beauty that every moment holds. You will once again become conscious of your spirit connection, allowing you to unfold your gifts. Life will seem like a beautiful and glorious dance, flowing with ease and a newly gained sense of trust in the present.

MUSTARD

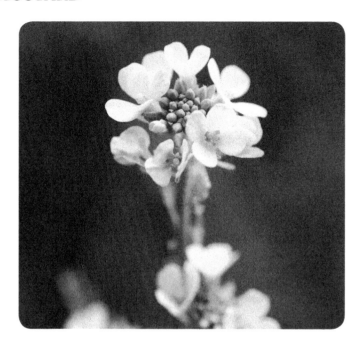

MESSAGE: I, Mustard, am bringing sunshine into your life, absorbing all feelings of despair and hopelessness, lifting your spirit while creating a strong connection to the vibration of universal love.

FOCUS: Flow of vitality – Hope – Trust – Light

CATEGORY: Staying focused in the present in all that you know – *Insufficient interest in present circumstances*

CHAKRAS: 2, 5, 7

COLOURS: White – Violet – Green

NUMBER: 33

When peace and harmony radiate within our being, we feel at ease; we live with joy and focus on the positive aspects of life and ourselves. There are times when it feels like a dark cloud is hanging over us, suppressing this joyful energy and lightness within us, creating disharmony and sadness. These limiting feelings may be caused by events from the past, including past lives, and the present, and may create blockages in the free flow of your life force. You frequently experience this sense of darkness resulting in a sense of heaviness, lack of vitality and motivation to enjoy life to its fullest. You may not know or understand why you are feeling this gloom and doom that causes feelings of hopelessness and helplessness.

With the support of Mustard strength and optimism will return. Mustard will assist you in moving the feeling of heaviness to the light, lifting your spirit and encouraging the light within to shine vibrant and strong. The essence of Mustard supports you in opening and clearing your connection to spirit, setting you free from limitations. You will experience a strong sense of knowing your spirit. With the help of Mustard joy, peace and happiness will become an integral part of your daily life, allowing you to see the beauty and opportunities for growth in any given moment. You will learn to listen to your higher self with your feelings, giving you recognition, strength and a strong sense of self-worth.

OLIVE

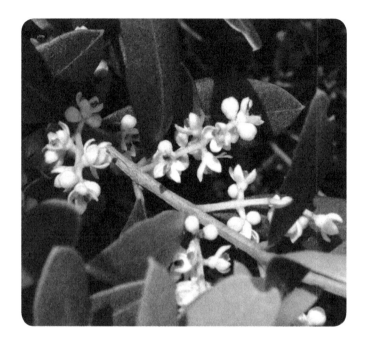

MESSAGE: I am Olive, the fountain of youth, restoring
            vitality on all levels of your being, while
            creating peace and harmony.

FOCUS: Strength – Harmony – Vitality – Peace

CATEGORY: Staying focused in the present in all
            that you know – *Insufficient interest in
            present circumstances*

CHAKRAS: 2, 4, 8 (thymus)

COLOURS: Yellow – Silver – Blue – Green

NUMBER: 29

Presently you are overcome by a feeling of exhaustion in all aspects of your life. Challenges of the past have drained you of your vitality affecting your physical, mental, emotional and spiritual stamina and balance. You may not be conscious of what it is that has created this state of depletion; however, you know that living your life right now requires great effort and that it lacks the natural flow. At times it feels like you have nothing left to give and cannot continue.

Olive is here to support you by reopening and clearing the channels that connect you to the Divine. Soon the energy will flow freely again, giving you strength, courage and stamina to continue on your path. You will once again be in harmony with life, experiencing a sense of trust, self-worth and spiritual knowing. With the help of Olive you will integrate the movement of frequencies from different dimensions easily. The compassionate and powerful nature of Olive will gently nourish your being on all levels, bringing back your energy and strength in a subtle yet profound way.

WHITE CHESTNUT

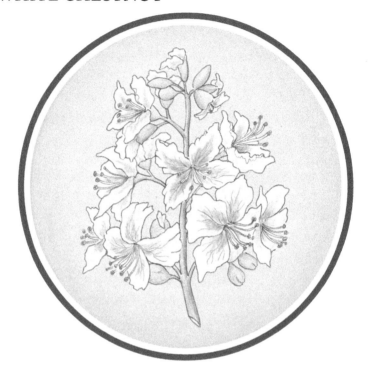

MESSAGE: I, White Chestnut, bring forth a magnificent
                light to fill your being. Breathe in this light
                and like a gentle breeze it will cleanse your
                mind, creating focus and peace of mind.

FOCUS: Focus – Clarity of mind – Peace
                – Centeredness

CATEGORY: Staying focused in the present in all
                that you know – *Insufficient interest in
                present circumstances*

CHAKRAS: 1, 7

COLOURS: White – Indigo – Gold – Lime green

NUMBER: 4

Our mind is powerful beyond imagination. It can have a very positive influence on creating and enhancing our life experiences. However, when it is filled with unwanted, undesirable and limiting thoughts, ideas and "conversations" it may become one of our biggest challenges. You are currently experiencing this type of situation where undesirable thoughts are constantly circling in your mind, interfering with your focus, clarity of mind and inner peace. Regardless of your efforts to change the situation the thoughts keep resurfacing. As a result life does not unfold easily, at times creating a sense of frustration and heaviness in body, mind and spirit.

White Chestnut has a very light and gentle nature bringing forth the energy of the sun, the source of life. The light energy will illuminate your being, clearing your mind of all its undesirable and limiting thoughts. You will gain clarity, allowing you to focus on the present and what it is you need to do. Your intuitive senses will be enlightened and you will be living your life with ease, in synchronized balance; thinking and speaking nothing but the highest truth.

WILD ROSE

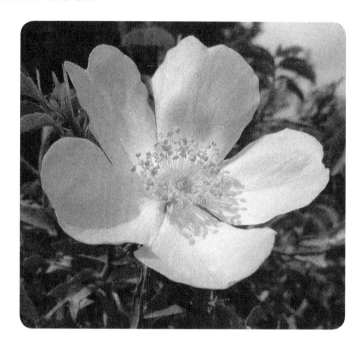

MESSAGE: I am Wild Rose, opening your heart, bringing
joy and awareness, guiding you to feel and
know that deep within you is what brings joy.

FOCUS: Love – Motivation – Awareness – Activation
of joy

CATEGORY: Staying focused in the present in all
that you know – *Insufficient interest in
present circumstances*

CHAKRAS: 1, 4, 6

COLOURS: Pink – Pearl – Indigo – White

NUMBER: 17

At times life simply moves on without us as an active player. The less we get actively and consciously involved in creating our own reality, the less interesting and exciting life appears to be. Truly experiencing joy in its deepest and life enriching meaning has slipped away from you. You have surrendered to the idea that life is taking its own course, not unfolding to your heart's desires. You may not even be aware anymore of your true spiritual essence and therefore what it is that you desire. As a result most aspects of your life have currently lost a sense of joy, love and synchronized balance – for self and others.

Wild Rose guides you to once again connect to your true spiritual essence which will fill your being with the pure essence of joy, love and light. You will feel joy return into every aspect of your life, motivating you to live your life consciously with softness and gentleness every step of the way. Wild Rose embraces you ever so gently and raises your vibrational frequencies so that you will regain clarity and understanding of your heart's desires. You will once again trust in your inner knowing and become the conscious creator of your life. With love and joy in your heart your life will unfold with great excitement and once again become a rewarding experience.

REFLECTIONS

CATEGORY 4:

- Nurture and Support Sense of Trust and Belonging – *Loneliness*
- Flowers: **Heather, Impatiens, Water Violet**

HEATHER

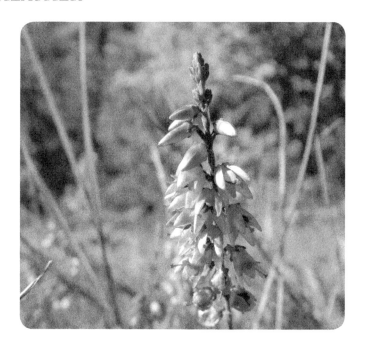

MESSAGE: I, Heather, am strengthening your connection to your true Soul essence, creating a sense of peace and comfort within yourself.

FOCUS: Increased sensibility towards self and others – Sense of belonging

CATEGORY: Nurture and support sense of trust and belonging – *Loneliness*

CHAKRAS: 1, 2, 5

COLOURS: Pink – Violet – Pearl – Blue

NUMBER: 3

Being alone and being lonely are two different things. We may be alone and truly enjoy our own company or we may feel lonely either when alone or even when being in company of others. You often feel lonely, finding it difficult to spend any length of time by yourself. Your need to share your "life" with others, regardless of who it might be, is intense. It seems like you lack the clear connection to your Soul essence which provides a sense of belonging and self-worth.

Your strong need for sharing may also interfere with honestly listening to and hearing what others wish to share, increasing your sense of loneliness even more.

Heather fills your being with love and kindness, supporting and comforting you. Your sense of loneliness and strong need to share with anyone who may be around will shift to an understanding and knowing within you, giving rise to new levels of self-worth. Heather guides you to listen with your feelings to your own needs and those of others, creating opportunities for mutual sharing and communication. With increased sensibility towards self and others you will feel a strong connection to your Soul and experience deepened levels of love, peace and harmony, making it easy to be alone without feeling lonely. You will flourish and shine, radiating strength with softness and kindness from your heart so that others will enjoy being around you.

IMPATIENS

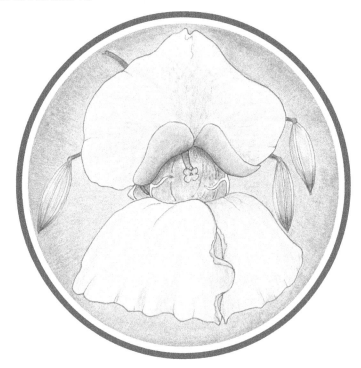

MESSAGE: Open your heart to all aspects of all life
within and around you. I, Impatiens, will
then flow through you, creating vibrations of
understanding and patience leading to peace
and harmony.

FOCUS: Acceptance – Perception – Patience

CATEGORY: Nurture and support sense of trust and
belonging – *Loneliness*

CHAKRAS: 3, 4, 7

COLOURS: Green – Yellow – White

NUMBER: 18

When we are filled with loving light for ourselves and others and we trust the process of life it is easy to be patient and kind at all times. Your nature is warm and friendly and you have great knowledge and a strong character. However, you get easily irritated when life does not present itself in a way you perceive to be right or when things move along too slowly. This lack of patience and acceptance creates tension and restlessness for yourself and others, leading to vibrations of disharmony in all aspects of your being – mental, spiritual, emotional and physical. Life does not flow as easily, effortlessly and effectively as it potentially could.

Impatiens nurtures you with an energy that brings calmness, patience and acceptance, assisting you in being loving and kind to yourself and others. You will experience a new sense of understanding, awareness and trust. Vibrations of disharmony and irritation will be washed away, creating space for balance, peace and harmony. Impatiens reminds you of your connection to spirit, the universal life force and Mother Earth, helping you to stay grounded in the physical world. With trust and clear focus in all that you know you will radiate patience and acceptance, touching many people's lives in a very calm, supportive and peaceful way.

WATER VIOLET

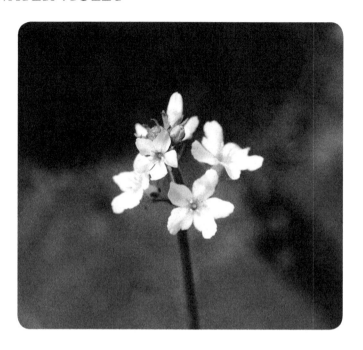

MESSAGE:	High frequencies resonate like soft music within you creating peace, harmony and a sense of belonging. This song, I share with you freely. Open your heart and "listen" carefully so that you may receive my healing vibrations.
FOCUS:	Synchronized harmony – Acceptance – Belonging
CATEGORY:	Nurture and support sense of trust and belonging – *Loneliness*
CHAKRAS:	3, 7
COLOURS	Violet – White – Gold – Blue-green translucent
NUMBER	9

Feelings of peace and harmony within fill our being with beauty and light giving us the strength and confidence to deal with life as it presents itself. The better we know ourselves, the easier it is to follow our personal direction with clarity and confidence. This awareness brings you strength and comfort. You are a very gentle, quiet person, generally feeling content being by yourself. You prefer moving around unnoticed, be it in everyday life or in more challenging times such as illness. Presently you are feeling off balance, experiencing a sense of loneliness. You have lost your usually clear and strong connection to spirit. You also recognize that you are different from others, leaving you at times with feelings of sadness and loneliness.

Water Violet, like yourself, has a very gentle and kind nature; it is vibrating peacefully at high frequencies. These vibrations will assist you in connecting to your deep spiritual knowing, allowing your intuition to once again flow freely and easily. The soft music of Water Violet will transform any feelings of sadness and disharmony into love and light. Inner peace and strength will return. Water Violet brings clarity, helping you to understand and accept why you are different from others. You will feel comfortable within yourself and spread light, peace and harmony wherever you go.

REFLECTIONS

CATEGORY 5:

- Strength to Stay Focused and True to One's Own Ideals - *Over-Sensitivity to Influences and Ideas from Others*
- Flowers: ***Agrimony, Centaury, Holly, Walnut***

AGRIMONY

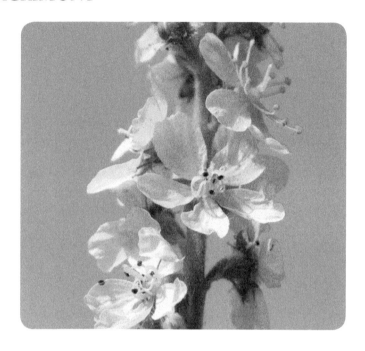

MESSAGE: I, Agrimony, fill your being with a bright light giving you the courage to be true to yourself and speak your truth.

FOCUS: Speaking and expressing your truth with confidence

CATEGORY: Strength to stay focused and true to one's own ideals – *Over-sensitivity to influences and ideas from others*

CHAKRAS: 2, 3, 6

COLOURS: Violet – Blue – White – Gold

NUMBER: 14

When peace and harmony are present in our lives we feel comfortable and joyful. We strive for love and acceptance from others but equally important is self-acceptance in all who we are. You have a strong need for peace and harmony but lack confidence. Acceptance and recognition from others are especially important to you. You have the tendency to avoid conflict, not speaking or expressing your truth; staying focused in all that you know is difficult. You show yourself as a joyful, easy-going person hiding deep inside your true feelings of unhappiness, distress and disagreement. Lack of self-worth and the denial of spiritual knowing create feelings of vulnerability and inadequacy.

Agrimony brings clarity and consciousness to you, giving you the courage and confidence required to follow your inner guidance. Like a flower in the budding stage you will open when the time is right and show your beauty and truth with confidence. Agrimony helps you to understand that your feelings, and what you know are of great value, and therefore guides you gently in situations of conflict. You will feel a new sense of connection to the Earth, giving you the strength and courage to stay true to your being. Sharing your innate nature with others will fill you with much joy, creating lightness that radiates outwards in a most beautiful vibrant golden light. Expressing what you know will build your confidence and set you free.

CENTAURY

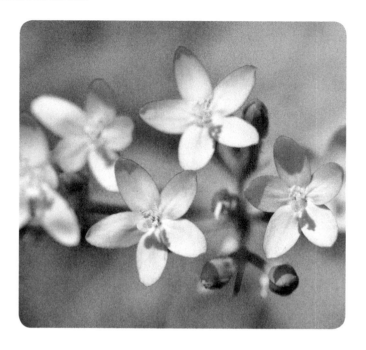

MESSAGE: Soft and gentle I, Centaury, impart trust and
                courage in you so that giving and receiving
                are a constant balance of ebb and flow like the
                waves of the ocean come and go.

FOCUS: Acceptance and recognition of self – Balance
                in giving and receiving

CATEGORY: Strength to stay focused and true to one's own
                ideals – *Over-sensitivity to influences and ideas*
                from others

CHAKRAS: 2, 3, 7

COLOURS: Pink – White – Pearl – Blue

NUMBER: 10

Life is like a story of balance created by the continuous flow of duality. For example: there is light and there is darkness, peace and war, happiness and sadness, synchronized balance and destruction, love and hate, well-being and dis-ease. Giving and receiving are an integral part of this duality and play a vital role in our journey on this planet. You have a very kind and gentle Soul, radiating softness and generosity, always caring for the well-being of others. However, maintaining the balance between giving and receiving can be a challenge for you because of your willingness to always lend a helping hand and your difficulty saying "no" when asked for assistance. As a result, you are at times being led astray from your purpose in life, not nurturing your own Soul sufficiently. Neglecting the direction of your own Soul causes you to feel tired, exhausted and overwhelmed.

Centaury is of very soft and caring vibrational frequencies and shares those freely with you, supporting you in recognizing your true Soul essence and encouraging you to live your life in accordance with it. Giving and receiving will begin to follow a balanced flow like leaves waving gently back and forth in a breeze. With increased consciousness you will learn to feel and know who you are, creating a balanced playing field of caring for others and your own personal needs. Universal love will flow freely into and within you, nurturing all levels of your being and giving you renewed strength and vitality.

Note: The higher vibrational frequencies of Mother Earth are changing the significance of giving and receiving; more now than ever before do we receive through giving and we give through receiving.

HOLLY

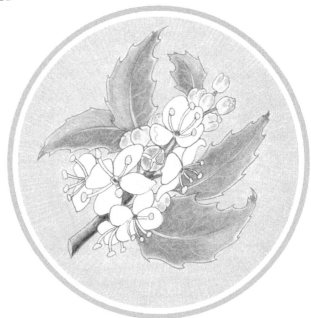

MESSAGE: Breathe deeply; open your heart and trust. Give yourself permission to feel and be filled with my energies of unconditional love so that every cell of your being radiates golden light, reflecting acceptance and understanding. Be gentle and loving to self and others.

FOCUS: Seeing and experiencing life through your heart – Gentleness – Love for self and others

CATEGORY: Strength to stay focused and true to one's own ideals – *Over-sensitivity to influences and ideas from others*

CHAKRAS: 1, 5, 7, 8 (thymus)

COLOURS: Turquoise – Pearl – White – Pink

NUMBER: 11

Love and light are essential to all life on this planet. Lack of either one of them affects the quality of life in all aspects – physical, mental, emotional and spiritual. Presently you are experiencing emotions such as heartaches, resentment, irritability, jealously, anger or sadness either towards yourself or others. The vibrational density of these emotions does not serve you, any other person or life form. The strong sense of unhappiness that has overcome you creates disharmony and disrupts the gentle and easy flow of the life force that nourishes and nurtures us.

Holly spreads love and joy unconditionally, creating harmonious vibrations within you. These high frequencies allow you to truly <u>feel</u> and accept the power of unconditional love. Experiencing love for self assists you in understanding that it is a prerequisite for loving others. Any self-defeating and destructive thoughts and feelings will be transformed into vibrations of gentleness, acceptance and understanding. You once again will become an open channel for the universal life force which creates a natural flow of giving and receiving, nourishing yourself, everyone and everything else around you. Holly reminds you that love and synchronized balance are the greatest healers of all.

WALNUT

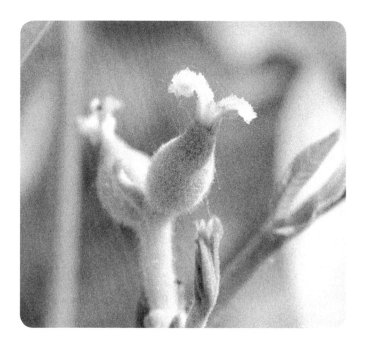

MESSAGE:	I, Walnut, illuminate the golden light within you, bringing clarity to your Soul purpose and giving you the strength and determination to be who you are regardless of outside influences. Unfold to your potential and be true to yourself.
FOCUS:	Clear vision of self – Transformation – Determination – Soul purpose
CATEGORY:	Strength to stay focused and true to one's own ideals – *Over-sensitivity to influences and ideas from others*
CHAKRAS:	2, 6, 7
COLOURS:	Gold – Blue – Yellow – White
NUMBER:	30

Every one of us is born with a directional focus in life yet very few of us are conscious of what this is. In general, you have a clear sense of your ideals and ambitions and strive to live in accordance with them. However, outside influences are causing restrictions and deviation from your ambitions in life and are interfering with your personal growth and your ability to live in harmony with your Soul. Are you wondering at times: Who am I? It feels like you are living in a cocoon that was not spun by yourself. It is time to break out of this cocoon so that you may transform into your own beauty and all that you are, leaving behind outside influences and restrictions that do not serve you.

Walnut assists you to live your life in truth and harmony with your Soul essence, creating clarity and a sense of fulfillment. It reminds you of your infinite source, reopening channels to bring consciousness to and awareness of your beautiful spirit. You will spread your wings and soar to new heights, leaving restrictions and outside influences behind. Discovering new shores and dimensions will lead to profound and rewarding transformation. Walnut whispers gently and lovingly: Always follow what resonates true to you in your heart. Move forward with courage and ease and leave behind any restrictions that were not spun by you.

REFLECTIONS

CATEGORY 6:

- Encouragement and Contentment with Heightened Capacity for Spiritual Knowledge – *Despondency and Despair*
- Flowers: **Crab Apple, Elm, Larch, Oak, Pine, Star of Bethlehem, Sweet Chestnut, Willow**

CRAB APPLE

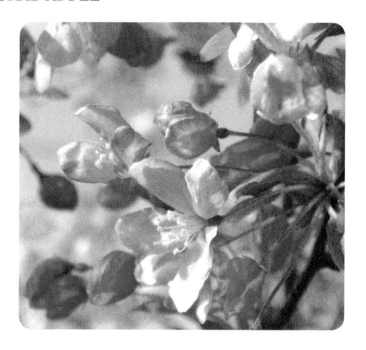

MESSAGE: I, Crab Apple, cleanse all levels of your
                  being by radiating the essence of light and
                  synchronized balance inside of you, allowing
                  you to shift your focus, embrace who you are
                  and heal.

FOCUS: Shifting focus – Cleansing – Lightness

CATEGORY: Encouragement and contentment with
                  heightened capacity for spiritual knowledge –
                  Despondency and despair

CHAKRAS: 1, 4, 7, 8 (thymus)

COLOURS: White – Gold – Green – Fuchsia

NUMBER: 27

Cleansing is a most vital element in all aspects of life on this planet; be it the cleansing of impurities of our physical body, our mind, our emotions or our spirit. So is Mother Earth in great need of cleansing right now. You are aware of the importance and benefits of cleansing but you have lost the balance in your focus. Minor impurities or imbalances within yourself, or life in general, may cause you distress and distract you from what is truly essential. You have lost sight of the ever present beauty, of yourself and/or all of life, leading you astray from the true essence of life.

Crab Apple assists you in cleansing your entire being, freeing your mind from being preoccupied and fixated on impurities according to your own perception. Your focus can now shift from small segments of life to all there is, allowing you to see and feel its entire beauty. This new perception creates an environment within and around you that is of lightness and acceptance, supporting cleansing and healing. Acceptance of self, of others and of circumstances will become natural and as a result you will radiate beauty in harmony, transforming lives including your own.

ELM

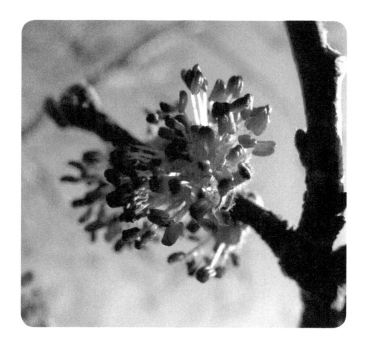

MESSAGE: With synchronized balance, I, Elm, open
your channels to the universe to all there is,
so that you are able to continue living your
Soul essence with courage, optimism, strength
and ease. Remember to breathe consciously
and deeply.

FOCUS: Living your truth – Optimism – Ease

CATEGORY: Encouragement and contentment with
heightened capacity for spiritual knowledge –
Despondency and despair

CHAKRAS: 1, 2, 7

COLOURS: Blue – White – Indigo – Pearl

NUMBER: 33

Your sense of responsibility and commitment to your Soul are strong. You are an open channel for the light coming into you, the light that guides you to live your true spiritual essence. This allows you to deal with many challenges simultaneously. However, right now you are feeling overwhelmed and distracted with the magnitude of responsibilities presenting themselves in your life. It seems like too many events and energies are coming at you, causing you to lose your centre and your usually strong sense of connectedness and purpose. This leads to restrictions in the free flow of the universal life force, creating moments of doubt about your own abilities and your willingness to continue your journey of light.

Elm is here to support you. Her vibrations fill you with renewed strength and optimism so that you will be able to continue to follow your purpose in life. Feelings of being overwhelmed will subside and be replaced with strength and knowing from deep within. Your motivation will return and lighter energies will once again flow freely through you, guiding you to accomplish all you have set out to do with synchronized balance – easily, effortlessly and effectively. You will shift your perception so that you can see the diversity of your tasks as opportunities for growth rather than as too many challenges. Stay connected to the Earth and your heart and Elm will show you how to live your truth in harmony with your Soul essence.

LARCH

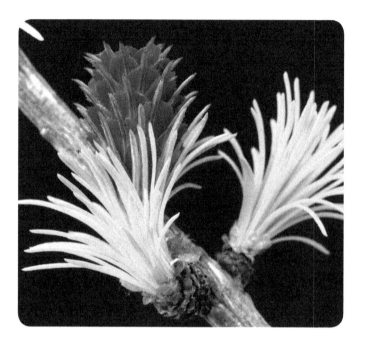

MESSAGE: I, Larch, am here to support you. Trust your inner beauty and abilities and you will discover new shores. Reach for the stars and the moon and watch yourself soar, unfolding to all you can and are meant to be.

FOCUS: Self-acceptance – Courage – Self-worth – Joy

CATEGORY: Encouragement and contentment with heightened capacity for spiritual knowledge – *Despondency and despair*

CHAKRAS: 1, 2, 8 (thymus)

COLOURS: Silver – Purple – Green

NUMBER: 28

Every one of us is special in our own right and we are all blessed with gifts unique to each one of us that are worth sharing. You are uncertain of your own abilities and gifts, often dealing with the feeling of lack of self-worth. You tend to compare yourself with others and believe that others around you are more capable and worthy than you are. This perception of yourself creates the anticipation of failure along with insecurities, uncertainty, uneasiness and occasional fear. As a result, you are holding back from unfolding your own gifts and potential, not moving forward with ease and becoming all who you are in your entire beauty.

Larch is here to assist you, guiding and supporting you on your journey on this Earth. Larch will open new doors, setting you free from your limiting beliefs about yourself, helping you to recognize and acknowledge your own unique gifts and beauty. Your connection to spirit will be strengthened and flow more freely and easily, giving you a clear sense of truth and spiritual knowing. The loving vibrations of Larch raise your spirits, offering courage and support so that you may develop a strong sense of self-worth and self-acceptance. Inner peace and trust will prevail. Life will bring great joy and you will move forward with ease, "standing tall" and knowing that, yes, you are capable and worthy like anyone sharing this journey with you.

OAK

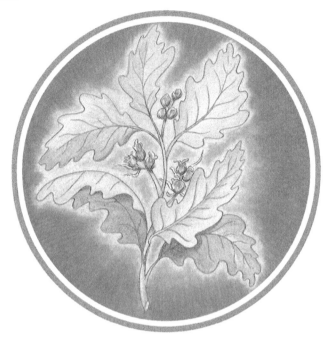

MESSAGE: We, the flowers of the Divine Oak, immerse
every cell of your being with our essence,
allowing you to feel the power and strength that
is inherent to gentleness. Always remember that
unconditional love in the form of synchronized
balance is the strongest healer of all.

FOCUS: Gentle strength – Kindness

CATEGORY: Encouragement and contentment with
heightened capacity for spiritual knowledge –
Despondency and despair

CHAKRAS: 1, 3

COLOURS: Green – Indigo – Violet – Gold

NUMBER: 7

The planet is changing and shifting into new dimensions and frequencies and at the same time Mother Earth is dealing with many challenges relating to her survival. Consequently, human-kind faces more, and different, demands than in the past. It is of great importance, now more than ever, to be strong within ourselves and to keep our connection to spirit open and free flowing in order to have the stamina to continue our mission as beings of light. You have great strength, stamina and determination, always continuing to improve and find solutions regardless of how hopeless a situation may seem. However, at times you get discouraged when things interfere with achieving your goals. Right now your struggles are intensified and solutions do not fall into place easily making life more difficult than usual. Your strength and determination are waning.

Oak shares her gentle strength and kindness freely with you and walks by your side as a teacher and friend. You will learn to understand that your strong determination to never give up may create resistance; a resistance that interferes with your light connection to the universal love energy, creating lack of vitality and possibly feelings of desperation and despair. Oak teaches you that we receive the greatest strength from true love and gentleness. The essence will guide you to recognize the softness and gentle-ness that is within you; this will then become the source of your strength and determination. Your spirit connection will be strong and flow with clarity, creating a life that unfolds effortlessly.

PINE

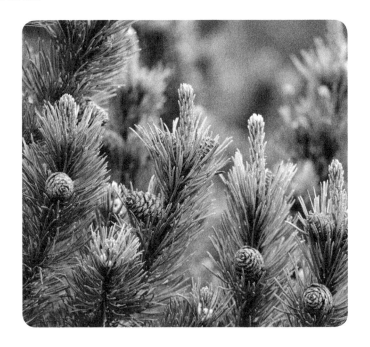

MESSAGE:	You were born to manifest the glory of the universe that is within you. Open your heart and you shall receive and understand that perfection is a perception.
FOCUS:	Gentleness – Gratitude – Perception – Confidence – Acceptance
CATEGORY:	Encouragement and contentment with heightened capacity for spiritual knowledge – *Despondency and despair*
CHAKRAS:	1, 3, 7, 8 (thymus)
COLOURS:	Gold – White – Blue – Pearl
NUMBER:	25

Being truly satisfied and seeing the value in one's own accomplishments creates feelings of joy and happiness. We are encouraged to continue to grow, and face new opportunities and challenges with confidence, love and light in our heart, mind and spirit. You have a strong desire to "shine" but are seldom content with your own achievements because you tend to focus on imperfections. You take responsibility for any mistakes even if they were not caused by yourself. This unjustified criticism weighs heavily on you, causing lack of confidence, influencing your actions and choices and hindering you from unfolding your skills and gifts in life.

Pine fills your being with gentleness and loving kindness. It helps you to remember that you are a child of the loving universe and that we are all equal. With the help of Pine your perception about yourself will shift, bringing clarity and confidence as the energy of highest truth will flow clearly and freely through you. Pine encourages you to be gentle with yourself and learn to accept your right to be brilliant, gorgeous and talented and to acknowledge your accomplishments as perfect the way they are, despite any imperfections. You will experience a new level of gentleness towards yourself, lightening your energies and lifting any heaviness. You will understand that playing small does not serve the world. The glory of the universe is within every one of us and as you give yourself permission to shine, you allow other people to do the same.

STAR OF BETHLEHEM

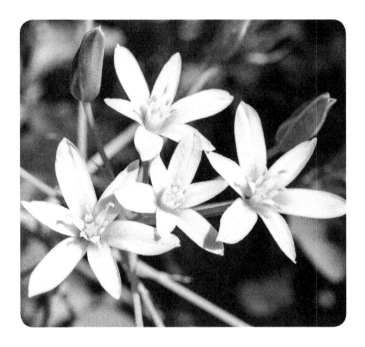

MESSAGE: I, Star of Bethlehem, fill your being with the most gentle and loving essence of hope and healing, releasing from your cellular memory all that does not serve you.

FOCUS: Healing – Release and integration of experiences into life – Peace

CATEGORY: Encouragement and contentment with heightened capacity for spiritual knowledge – *Despondency and despair*

CHAKRAS: 1, 3, 5, 7

COLOURS: White – Blue-green – Pink – Violet – Turquoise – Lime green – Pearl

NUMBER: 1

Life's experiences are stored in our cellular memory which may create blockages, interfering with the free flow of the universal energy. The cellular memory can hold us back from all we can be, creating disharmony and imbalances on the physical, mental, emotional and spiritual level. Some unresolved challenges or trauma (small or large) from the past, including past lives or the present, are affecting you right now. You feel hampered in your personal growth, lacking the ease with which you desire your life to flow.

Star of Bethlehem brings healing and comfort to you like no other and through its energies allows the release of the cellular memory that interferes with the creation of your life in accordance with your Soul essence. It ever so gently washes away all that is holding you "hostage" from any experiences, past or current. Wounds will heal, leading to new levels of awareness and possibilities. Peace and harmony will emanate from you, allowing the connection to your Soul to flow with ease. Star of Bethlehem guides you on your path to healing and encourages you to see the truth through feeling it and becoming at peace with it. You may get a sense of being "reborn", creating an environment for enhanced personal growth.

SWEET CHESTNUT

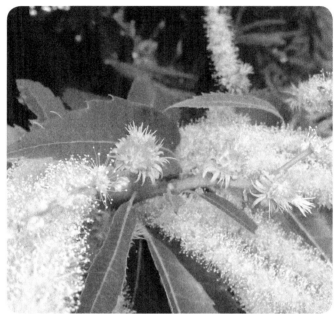

MESSAGE: I, Sweet Chestnut, enlighten your being, sharing my love and light freely with you. Take a deep breath, step back and relax so you can clearly see the light at the end of the tunnel.

FOCUS: Stamina – Breath of life – Light

CATEGORY: Encouragement and contentment with heightened capacity for spiritual knowledge – *Despondency and despair*

CHAKRAS: 1, 5, 6, 7

COLOURS: Gold – Pearl – Pink – White – Violet

NUMBER: 5

At times life presents itself with so many obstacles and challenges that it seems unbearable. These outside influences interfere with our connection to spirit and our ability to live life in accordance with our Soul essence. You are of a very sensitive nature, at the same time showing great strength. Presently, however, your load in life feels too heavy and you are being pushed beyond what you believe you are able to handle. Your inner strength is waning, making it difficult for you to continue on your path. Your consciousness of your Soul essence and spiritual knowing are being overshadowed by feelings of despair. Your inner light has lost its strength to shine, enlighten and nourish all aspects of your being.

Sweet Chestnut comes forward with softness, sharing the breath of life with you freely and lovingly. Once again your inner light will shine bright and strong, enlightening your being and encouraging you to clearly see the beauty of life and feel the support of the universe. As your light becomes stronger, so will your connection to spirit, bringing back stamina and vitality and the desire to continue to follow your Soul's guidance. Sweet Chestnut supports you in finding your light, balance and inner strength and shifting your focus from the dark to the light sides of life. The light within you will regain a vibrant glow, radiating balance and harmony helping to spread Light on Earth.

WILLOW

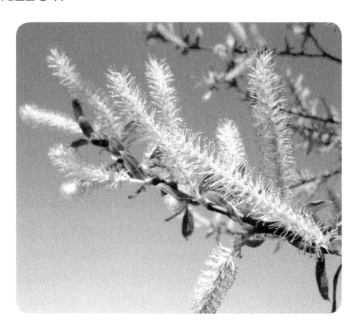

MESSAGE: I, Willow, flood you with synchronized harmony, cleansing all that is not yours and teach you the true meaning of "master of your own destiny". I spark a bright light within you empowering you to live your life energized with passion and intent.

FOCUS: Master of own destiny – Ambition – Motivation

CATEGORY: Encouragement and contentment with heightened capacity for spiritual knowledge – *Despondency and despair*

CHAKRAS: 1, 3, 5

COLOURS: Green – Indigo – Green-blue – Blue – White – Pearl

NUMBER: 23

At times life presents itself with continuous challenges and set-backs and it may seem like more things are going wrong in your own life than in other people's lives around you. You feel like a victim of your circumstances, looking for reasons for this "injus-tice" outside of yourself. With it you may harbour feelings of anger, resentment and bitterness; all creating a lack of the flow of vital life force. When "things go wrong" according to your own perception you have the tendency to withdraw yourself and lose motivation to pursue your goals and ideals. Physical imbalances are imminent.

Willow supports you through tough times, filling you with synchronized balance and clarity. With softness the essence gives you the strength to shake off outside influences easily and to continue on your path. You will comprehend that adverse circumstances are not sufficient reason to withdraw yourself as the victim. Willow brings encouragement and strength to make it easier for you to take responsibility. This will soften your energies and keep you motivated to live your life according to your Soul essence. Willow shares her gift with you freely and uncondition-ally. Accept with gratitude and an open heart and you will become the master of your own destiny!

REFLECTIONS

CATEGORY 7:

- Living in Synchronized Balance and Understanding of the Highest (Heart Woven) Truth – *Over-Care for Welfare of Others*
- <u>Flowers:</u> *Beech, Chicory, Rock Water, Vervain, Vine*

BEECH

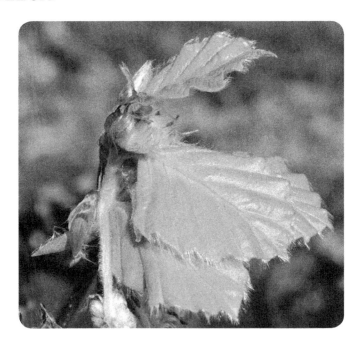

MESSAGE: I, Beech, encourage you to open your heart to my spirit so that you may receive and understand the beauty of acceptance with softness and kindness in all creation within and around you.

FOCUS: Individuality – Gentleness – Acceptance

CATEGORY: Living in synchronized balance and understanding of the highest (heart woven) truth – *Over-care for welfare of others*

CHAKRAS: 1, 4, 7

COLOURS: Silver – White – Lime green – Fuchsia – Turquoise

NUMBER: 21

Wherever we look in this world today we see disharmony created by disrespect and lack of acceptance and understanding for Mother Earth and humankind. Peace on Earth as well as within us are only possible when we follow the guidance of our Soul which means walking this sacred land with reverence, love, acceptance and tolerance every step of the way. You tend to criticize yourself, not seeing your own beauty and gifts. Lack of self-respect and acceptance might make it difficult for you to accept others as individuals on their own journey, not allowing you to see the beauty and diversity in all there is.

Beech asks you to open your heart and listen with your feelings to its spirit song. Your wonderful being will be filled with loving light, softening your energies towards yourself and others. Every single cell will vibrate in synchronized balance, transforming criticism, disrespect and lack of understanding to acceptance and respect. Beech teaches you how to embrace life with a positive, nurturing outlook rather than looking for faults and imperfections. You will truly understand and be able to accept that as individuals we are at different stages in our lives and move through life accordingly. With renewed trust and realization of your own inner truth you will blossom and shine.

CHICORY

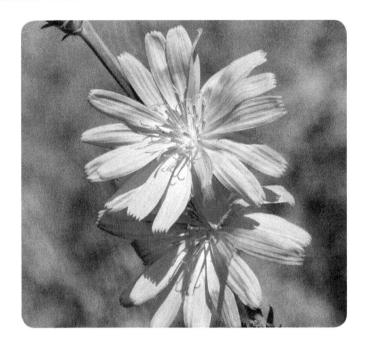

MESSAGE:	I, Chicory, fill your energy fields–physical, emotional, esoteric–with my magical, iridescent blue light so that you may experience happiness, peace and harmony arising from within you.
FOCUS:	Balance between giving and receiving – Contentment within self – Respect for others
CATEGORY:	Living in synchronized balance and understanding of the highest (heart woven) truth – *Over-care for welfare of others*
CHAKRAS:	1, 7
COLOURS:	Blue – White – Pink
NUMBER:	8

Truly and deeply caring for others with love is a precious quality and desperately needed for the survival of humankind and the planet. You have a strong need to assist family, friends and others under any circumstances. You have the tendency to impose your ideas assuming that what you know is best for others. As a result, your caring nature may create interference and dependency. You also wish for the people you care for to be close to you. Your desire to lend a helping hand and give advice at all times is not always received in the way you believe it should be. You may feel disappointed, disheartened, unappreciated and unloved.

Chicory will flood your energy fields with a magnificent, iridescent blue light creating peace and harmony within you and bringing clarity to your spirit connection. Vibrations of synchronized balance, love for self and others will flow through you easily and effortlessly. You will learn to recognize when advice and assistance are appropriate and when to keep to yourself. Chicory allows you to experience a new sense of balance, supporting you in providing comfort and clarity to anyone, humankind, animal and plant, without interfering with personal choice and freedom.

ROCK WATER

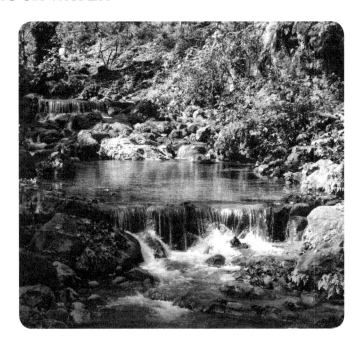

MESSAGE: I, Rock Water, am the spring of life. "Listen" to me with your heart and follow my guidance so your life will flow with ease like a gentle flowing river, seeing the beauty and joy in every moment of life.

FOCUS: Going with the flow – Flexibility – Grounding – Rebirthing

CATEGORY: Living in synchronized balance and understanding of the highest (heart woven) truth – *Over-care for welfare of others*

CHAKRAS: 1, 2, 7

COLOURS: Blue – Aquamarine – Violet – Gold

NUMBER: 31

Rock Water is continuously and joyfully bubbling from a healing spring, creating new moments in a playful way. Life is a never ending creation of moments. As the water flows with ease, finding its path, so have we the choice to live our life like a flowing river, openly embracing the beauty, opportunities and challenges as they arise. You set high standards for yourself and in order to achieve your goals you tend to follow a straight path, not recognizing opportunities as they arise. Lack of flexibility and spontaneity interfere with listening to and following your inner truth and spiritual knowing. Following the guidance of your Soul can cause uneasiness because of your resistance to leave your comfort zone.

Rock Water, the source of life and healing, guides you to live your life with ease like a flowing river that is forever changing with moments of stillness for reflection without losing sight of your destiny. The playful and joyful nature of Rock Water encourages you to bring energies of softness and lightness into your daily life. Just like the spring is giving birth to Rock Water every single moment, so are you the creator of every moment in your own life. Rock Water deepens your levels of consciousness while at the same time ensuring that you are grounded. You will be able to live your life with increased flexibility, giving yourself permission to take detours or alter your goals as you flourish through your own experiences. Rock Water encourages you to embrace all that comes into your awareness and move with it like an ever changing river.

In addition, Rock Water assists anyone with the process of rebirthing.

VERVAIN

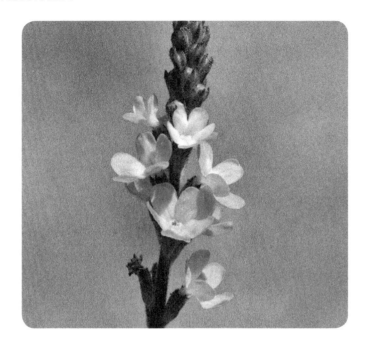

MESSAGE:	I, Vervain, fill your being with softness and kindness. I share with you the understanding that knowing your truth is a gift but that not everyone shares the same truth.
FOCUS:	Fairness – Truth – Acceptance – Surrender
CATEGORY:	Living in synchronized balance and understanding of the highest (heart woven) truth – *Over-care for welfare of others*
CHAKRAS:	1, 4, 7
COLOURS:	Violet – Blue – White – Turquoise – Gold
NUMBER:	35

Some of us have very clear and strong principles believing we know what is right or wrong. This creates a deep sense of justice. You have an exceptionally clear understanding of your truth. You feel easily disheartened with what you perceive as injustice. You have high standards and strive for perfection and excellence in every aspect of your life. You are experiencing disharmony and dissension within you, making you restless and easily irritable. You wish others around you would follow your standards, beliefs and principles. Your strong convictions create the desire within you to convince others to adopt your personal ideas and ideals.

Vervain is of a very kind and gentle nature, encouraging you to breathe deeply and softening your energy. It brings clarity, shifting any feelings of discouragement into vibrational frequencies of acceptance, love and understanding. In this world of injustice Vervain will nurture and support you, creating trust and strengthening your sense of belonging on this planet. The essence of Vervain encourages a gentle flow of energy within you, creating harmony and acceptance allowing your life to unfold with ease. Remember that knowing your truth is a gift but not everyone shares the same truth.

VINE

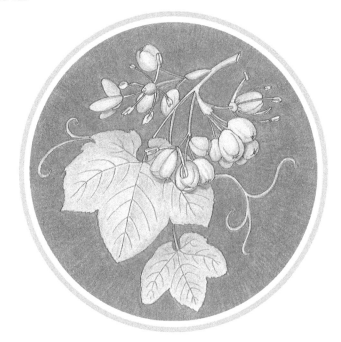

MESSAGE: Be strong but gentle and open your heart towards others, assisting them in seeing and understanding new levels of awareness and consciousness.

FOCUS: Flow with softness and gentleness – Observation – Leadership

CATEGORY: Living in synchronized balance and understanding of the highest (heart woven) truth – *Over-care for welfare of others*

CHAKRAS: 1, 2, 5, 8 (thymus)

COLOURS: Green – Blue – Pearl – Blue-green iridescent – Orange

NUMBER: 38

Every one of us is blessed with gifts that become part of our journey provided we choose to live according to our Soul essence. Even though you might not be aware of it, you are a born leader, giving you the ability to see, understand and assess situations clearly. You make decisions with confidence and it is natural for you to assist others and encourage them to take responsibility for their own journey. At times you find it challenging to accept and respect another person's actions and choices especially when they differ from what you perceive to be right or best. The desire or need to delegate or control creates vibrations of rigidity and restrictions, interfering with what you could potentially achieve. A competent leader is motivated through the heart and speaks nothing but the truth with love and kindness.

Vine helps you to recognize your innate leadership qualities and teaches you to reach out to others in a loving and under-standing way. Vine assists you in connecting to the softness of your Soul, allowing your strength and inner wisdom to radiate gently from you while asking your ego to step aside. Any wisdom shared in this manner will have the essence of pure love and is ultimately for the highest good of all–humankind and Mother Earth. Respect for and acceptance of others will follow easily and as a result others will clearly recognize the value of your leadership and move forward accordingly. Stay connected to your heart and you will speak and live nothing but the highest truth, becoming a true leader in support and healing of the Earth.

REFLECTIONS

RESCUE REMEDY

- Clarity and Strength for Inner Peace – *Stress and Trauma*
- <u>Flower Combination:</u> ***Clematis, Rock Rose, Cherry Plum, Impatiens, Star of Bethlehem***

RESCUE REMEDY

Clematis – Rock Rose – Cherry Plum – Impatiens – Star of Bethlehem

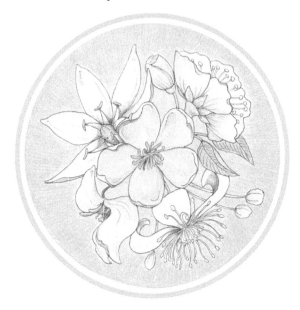

MESSAGE:	Breathe deeply and calmly and I will support you in restoring peace and harmony within you by filling your being with loving light.
FOCUS:	Universal intelligence – Calmness – Trust – Grounding – Courage – Healing
CATEGORY:	Clarity and strength for inner peace – *Stress and trauma*
CHAKRAS:	1, 3, 5, 6
COLOURS:	Turquoise – Gold – Pearl – Pink – White
NUMBER:	19

When all aspects of our life are in balance we can deal with adversities and challenges in an effective way, restoring peace and harmony without too much effort. However, at times the demands of life seem overwhelming and we lose our balance feeling lost, restless and maybe fearful. Unusual circumstances such as an accident, serious health issues or the loss of a loved one may cause us more stress than we believe we can handle. You are currently experiencing times of undue stress, wishing for better and easier times. This stress is affecting all aspects of your life–physical, mental, emotional and spiritual. It interferes with the free flow of the loving universal life force and with your ability to listen to it and follow its guidance. You have lost your balance and with it peace and harmony within you.

Rescue Remedy, a combination of five Bach Flowers vibrating in harmony, supports you during these stressful times. Regardless of how the stress manifests in you, Rescue Remedy brings instant relief and healing in all aspects required, assisting you in grounding and regaining your balance. It gives you the courage, strength, trust and confidence to truly deal with your experience(s) in the here and now. The healing vibrations of Rescue Remedy will clear any frequencies and energy blockages that might cause limitations and interfere with the free flow of Divine guidance. Rescue Remedy floods every part of your being with the infinite breath of life and beautiful light frequencies restoring balance, trust, peace and harmony.

REFLECTIONS

CHAPTER 10

Who Can Benefit
from Bach Flowers

"The amount of peace, of happiness, of joy, of health and of well-being that comes into our lives depends also on the amount of which the Divine Spark can enter and illuminate our existence. From time immemorial, man has looked at two great sources for Healing. To his Maker, and to the Herbs of the field, which his Maker has placed for the relief of those who suffer."
—EDWARD BACH

Bach Flower essences are extremely versatile and there is no limit to who could benefit from their use. Any living organism can potentially be supported in whichever way is needed at a given time. This includes all human beings, animals and plants regardless of age and condition.

BACH FLOWERS AND HUMANKIND

*"The prevention and cure of disease can be found by discovering
the wrong within ourselves and eradicating this fault by
the earnest development of the virtue which will destroy
it; not by fighting the wrong, but by bringing in such flood
of its opposing virtue that it will be swept from nature."*

—EDWARD BACH

The gentle nature of Bach Flower essences fills every cell of any living creature with nothing but positive virtues to raise the vibrational frequencies and thus encourage change, growth and healing. Consequently Bach Flower essences can be used safely by anyone including infants and pregnant women. Both can benefit greatly from taking the Bach Flower remedies, supporting them through transitional changes and emotional experiences throughout these times.

Every human being is an individual with their own unique personality and path to follow. Our personality is reflected by our mind which according to Dr. Bach is *"the most delicate and sensitive part of ourselves."* Since Bach Flowers address all possible states of mind and emotions and can do no harm, anyone will benefit from adding them to their "toolbox for life". Bach developed this system of healing so that it might serve as a gift from nature and the Divine to bring us closer to our Soul so that we may live free of limitations, unfold to our full potential and fulfill our purpose in life, whatever this may be.

BACH FLOWERS AND CHILDREN

"Parenthood is an office in life which passes from one to another, and is in essence a temporary giving of guidance and protection for a brief period, after which time it should then cease its efforts and leave the object of its attention free to advance alone."

—EDWARD BACH

The lives of children are in general very positive but there are times when emotions may interfere and Bach Flower remedies can help a child to deal with them in a positive and constructive way. Children experience many different developmental stages and situations in a short period of time and depending on their personality, their upbringing and life's circumstances they may feel challenged. They react according to their own character which shows in their behaviour and potentially the development of different dis-ease processes.

Some of the changes children need to cope with are for example, the arrival of a sibling, being in daycare, going to school, overcoming shyness or feelings of inadequacy, bullying (both being bullied and being a bully) and dissension in the parents' home.

Teenagers typically face their own set of challenges such as issues with self-image and identity, mood swings, onset of menstruation and physical changes during puberty.

Children are like sponges, prone to absorb other people's energies including thoughts and feelings. It is also common for well-meant family members, friends and teachers to impose their own ideas, ideals and expectations onto children – consciously or subconsciously. All of this creates challenges and interference for the children to stay connected to their Higher Self, possibly suppressing their development on many different levels including innate gifts. It is easy for them at such a delicate stage in their lives to lose sight of their own purpose and mission, and therefore the ability to live in accordance with their Soul.

If it is obvious that the energies of a child and parent or other family member are intertwined, it is beneficial for all involved to work with the Bach Flower essences. The simultaneous use of the remedies by different family members increases the likelihood of true healing.

Bach Flower remedies can help make any situation and transition in a child's life easier by providing support, filling and illuminating their delicate beings with the positive virtues of the loving flowers. As a result, they become stronger individuals with a clearer sense of who they are. This enables them to keep their channels of communication with their Higher Self free flowing, enabling them to trust their innate intuitive senses and ultimately be able to live their life in harmony with their Soul. When they do get sick, they will be able to recover more easily and quickly.

Administering the Bach Flower remedies for children is easy as well; they may be taken internally or externally. Even though the Bach Flower essences are preserved with brandy, the amount of alcohol in a treatment bottle is insignificant – two drops of each Bach Flower essence diluted with spring water in a 30ml (tincture) bottle. For more specifics see Chapter 11, *Practical Information.*

In my practice the children decorate their own treatment bottle with stickers. They are fond of their "brave medicine", "happy medicine" or whatever we may call it. Since no harm can be done, they are in charge of taking their own "potion" whenever they desire. This in itself is a very empowering experience for children. The only stipulation I have is that they sit down when they are taking the remedy directly from the bottle because the droppers I use are glass. This measure reduces the risk of injury from accidentally biting on the glass while being physically active.

Children typically respond more quickly to treatment because they carry less "baggage" and their connection to their Higher Self and Soul is more open than with most adults. They can be trusted in deciding when and how often to take their "potion" which includes respecting their decision to discontinue the use of a specific Bach Flower essence.

> *"The whole attitude of parents should be to give the little newcomer all the spiritual, mental and physical guidance to the utmost of their ability, ever remembering that the wee one is an individual soul come down to gain his own experience and knowledge in his own way according to the dictates of his Higher Self, and every possible freedom should be given for unhampered development."*
>
> **—EDWARD BACH**

BACH FLOWERS AND ANIMALS

Animals, just like human beings, are characterized by their own unique personality and will react to different situations according to their own temperament and mental state. They have emotions like human beings which include feelings of loneliness, jealousy, fear, anger, separation anxiety, happiness, excitement or depression.

For example, many animals are afraid of thunderstorms or going to the vet or groomer. In these cases a Bach Flower out of the first category that deals with fear may be indicated, giving the animal a sense of security.

Bach Flower remedies can be employed in the healing of all animals such as cats, dogs, horses, cows, birds and reptiles. The challenge is that animals do not use verbal language to communicate their emotions and so we need to rely on our observations and intuitive senses to assess a situation and choose the Bach Flower essences accordingly. Some people have the gift of communicating with animals in their own way but the reality is that this only applies to a minority of people.

When working with Bach Flowers and animals it is important to keep in mind that they also have the tendency to absorb energies from their owners and surroundings. Their health and emotions may be a reflection and expression of the owner's circumstances. It is common to see that pets have the same illnesses their owners deal with; this is something I have come across in my practice and teachings and has been confirmed by veterinarians. In such cases it is advisable to treat both the animal and owner with the Bach Flowers.

As with humans, it is important to consider the individual moods, emotions and behaviour of the respective animal when deciding on which remedies to use; the same behaviour may be the result of totally different emotions. For example, a dog may bark because they are afraid, aggressive or because they want to protect "their" territory and/or owner. Each situation suggests the use of a different Bach Flower even though the behaviour is the same.

An example for choosing a Bach Flower essence combination for an animal that has been moved to a new home environment could be: *Walnut* to assist in the change in the environment, *Honeysuckle* to encourage the animal to "be" in the present instead of "dwelling" on the past, *Wild Rose* to help the animal to see the joy in the new circumstances and *Rescue Remedy* to assist in dealing with any stress factors related to the move.

The choice of the remedy is obvious when shock and trauma are involved. These experiences are common for animals and call for the use of *Rescue Remedy*; often no subsequent treatment is required.

The application of the remedies for animals is easy. They can be added to their drinking water, their food, squirted into their mouth or applied externally. Rubbing them into the tips of the ears of dogs and cats and other large animals is a great way of administering the Bach Flower essences.

Following is one of Dr. Bach's case histories from 1935 for the use of Bach Flower essences with horses.

THE WHITE PONY

The farm hand said he was digging the grave for the pony for he was foaming at the mouth, had not eaten for some days and could hardly stand on his feet. They thought he would be dead within an hour or so.

Then the farm-hand said, Dr. Bach came along and said to him 'Can you hold his tongue to one side?' He did so, and the Doctor took a small bottle out of his pocket and poured it down the pony's throat.

He said to the farm-hand, "You can fill up the grave. Give the pony his usual food and drink" and went away.

The farm hand did as the Doctor said, the pony ate and drank and completely recovered.

The remedies given are unknown, probably Rock Rose or the Rescue Remedy.

- HOWARD, JUDY, AND JOHN RAMSELL

BACH FLOWERS AND PLANTS

*"The Story of the Oak Tree. (Oak is one of the Bach Flower
essences – author's note) One day, and not very long ago, a man
was leaning against an oak tree in an old park in Surrey, and he
heard what the oak tree was thinking."…. "And years afterwards
the man found that in the oak flowers of the oak tree was a great
power, the power to heal a lot of sick people, and so he collected
the flowers of the oak tree and made them into medicines, and
lots and lots of people were healed and made well again."*

—EDWARD BACH

Plants are living organisms that communicate in their own
unique ways, with each other and with human beings. They experience and express emotions and can be plagued with physical
disease. Therefore, plants too will respond favourably to treatment with Bach Flower essences.

Examples for the use of Bach Flower remedies with plants:

- Dis-eased plant: *Crab Apple* for the cleansing effect; *Star
  of Bethlehem* in case the dis-ease is related to some type of
  traumatic event.
- Neglected plants may become hopeless which indicates
  the use of *Gorse.*
- Re-potting or transplanting: *Star of Bethlehem* will
  help to overcome the trauma that might be associated
  with it and *Walnut* will make it easier to adjust to the
  new environment.

Rescue Remedy may be added to all the above cases to coun-
teract the element of stress that is part of each of the situations.

If you are not sure which Bach Flower essence to use or do not have any other than the *Rescue Remedy* on hand, you can simply work with the *Rescue Remedy*. More often than not you will see amazing and wonderful results.

CHAPTER 11

Practical Information

"No science, no knowledge is necessary, apart from the simple methods described herein; and they who will obtain the greatest benefit from this God-sent Gift will be those who keep it pure as it is; free from science, free from theories, for everything in nature is simple."

—EDWARD BACH

One of the wonderful aspects and great advantages of working with Bach Flower essences is that it is so simple and no prerequisites in regard to knowledge or understanding are needed. When Edward Bach was searching for this system of healing, his desire was to find a method that provided true healing, was simple to use and affordable for everyone.

This means every person from every walk of life can work with and benefit from these wondrous flower essences. Even though there are guidelines for using them, there is no need to complicate a simple process.

WHEN TO USE BACH FLOWERS

"So we see how great is the power of the right herbs to heal; not only to keep us strong and protect us from disease, not only to stop an illness when it is threatened, not only to relieve and cure us when we may be in distress and ill, but even to bring peace and happiness and joy to our minds when there is apparently nothing wrong with our health."

—EDWARD BACH

The above quote sums it up beautifully as to when the use of Bach Flower essences may be indicated. In short, whenever you feel like it. More specifically, when you have the need or desire for any kind of support or guidance. If you are dealing with an emotional, mental, spiritual or physical issue, a long-standing or acute situation, minor or major circumstances, the Bach Flowers have their place in a person's life provided one chooses to work with them.

The remedies encourage a person to get closer to one's Soul essence, making it easier to recognize one's intuition and follow the guidance of one's Higher Self. They not only empower an individual to take responsibility for their own well-being but in fact require the willingness to do so. An openness to change and transform limitations into positive attributes is also a prerequisite for healing.

Most commonly people will resort to the Bach Flowers when they are experiencing a crisis or are under stress; however, Bach Flower remedies are also a great preventative tool. For example, a person who tends to be fearful and plagued with anxiety may over time develop an ulcer or other health complications. If these emotional components (fear and anxiety) are being addressed and diminished, or even transformed with the help of Bach Flower essences, a physical crisis can potentially be averted.

Since healing and personal growth are lifelong processes Bach Flower essences may be used as companions for life. The decision about when to implement the essences is merely a personal choice.

Examples

There are no circumstances, emotional or mental states when the Bach Flower essences could not be found to be useful.

Prevention: Stress, mood fluctuations, daily ups and downs, anticipated situation triggering stress responses (interview, exam, dentist etc.)

> *"Prevention is better than cure, and these remedies help us in a wonderful way to get well, and to protect ourselves from attack of unpleasant things."*
>
> **—EDWARD BACH**

Acute and Chronic Dis-Ease: Any challenge – physical, mental, emotional and/or spiritual

> *"Never let anyone give up hope of getting well, such wonderful improvements and such marvelous recoveries have happened with the use of these herbs, even in those in which it was considered hopeless that anything could be done; that to despair is no longer necessary."*
>
> **—EDWARD BACH**

Support: Prior or during exams or interviews, decision making, when looking for guidance, any emotional/mental states such as fears, lack of focus, sense of loneliness.

Accidents: Acute care with _Rescue Remedy_

METHODS AND PRACTICAL GUIDELINES FOR SELECTING BACH FLOWERS

"Once we realise our own Divinity the rest is easy."

—EDWARD BACH

Edward Bach's medical career, including his research, laid the foundation for the creation of the method of healing with Bach Flowers. However, it was his strong connection to his spirit and to nature, his intuition and willingness to _"obey the commands of his Soul"_ (Edward Bach) that ultimately led him to the work with the flowers and plants. This means that using our intuition as a guide for choosing the flowers can be given high priority.

My experiences over 30 years, working with clients, friends and strangers in many parts of the world, have proven to me that the intuition is a reliable tool in choosing the appropriate flowers and of course the simplest method of all.

Even for those who have very little consciousness about their own spirit or connection to their Higher Self, choosing the relevant flowers by relying on their intuition has proven to be most accurate. The easiest tool for choosing the flowers this way is _Bach Flowers Unfolding,_ a deck of cards I created and published. Using our intuition works well for all ages, children and adults alike including those who are mentally challenged. See Chapter 16, _Bach Flowers Unfolding,_ for more details.

Relying on our intuition has another advantage worth mentioning. Our mind is very powerful and can be a wonderful tool but at the same time it can literally stand in the way of connecting to our subconscious, our Higher Self and our Soul. In this way the mind can create limitations, not allowing us to be consciously aware of what it is we really require in order to move forward in life. There are also times when we might choose not to look at the real issues. Life is complex and grasping it with our conscious mind alone only allows us to get glimpses of all there is.

Trusting our intuition, perhaps with the guidance of a competent and trustworthy person or friend, is a favorable way of choosing flower essences. We can rest assured that our intuition will only guide us to choose those flowers that relate to issues we are ready to acknowledge and work with. Relying on our intuition will often surprise us with entirely unexpected results but these are nevertheless truly amazing in the way that truth is being revealed.

"This work of healing has been done, and published and given freely so that people like yourselves can help yourselves"

—EDWARD BACH

Intuition

Take a few moments and deep breaths to focus your attention within before choosing a flower essence you are drawn to. You may choose a Bach Flower without thinking about anything in particular or you may want to focus on a specific question or situation for which you would like to receive guidance, support or healing.

Examples for general questions: Which flower is going to assist me the most in unfolding to my true and full potential? Which

Bach Flower will enhance my intuition or deepen the connection to my Soul?

Examples for specific questions: Which flower will assist me best with my current health issues, or in letting go of my children, or in preparing for the upcoming exam?

In my clinic, clients will pick a card from *Bach Flowers Unfolding* at the beginning of each year. The flower coming forward is an indication of what challenges may be awaiting a person at some point in the year ahead. The Bach Flower may not become relevant until much later in the year; however, the vibrational frequencies of the flower one is drawn to will on a subconscious level already "work" with a person's Higher Self, harmonizing the energies and in this way preparing the individual for what is to come.

One year a woman chose *Cherry Plum*, the Bach Flower for desperation, extreme fear and fear of losing one's mind. Later in the year the individual was diagnosed with cancer causing all the emotions to surface that *Cherry Plum* addresses. Even though the situation was not changed by the choice of *Cherry Plum*, the energetic support was there for her right from the beginning.

On another occasion, *Larch* was the flower of the year; *Larch* for lack of confidence and self-worth. The person was surprised and felt like she already had dealt with this challenge in her life and did not require *Larch* anymore. In the third quarter of the year, her career required her to step into a new arena of responsibilities with which she was very uncomfortable. All of a sudden, *Larch* became a great friend to help her overcome her lack of confidence and feelings of inferiority.

Some of my clients find comfort and support by choosing a Bach Flower for the following day (or week) at night before going to bed. This also allows the vibrational frequencies of the flower essence to harmonize with the vibrations of the individual throughout the night, creating a favourable environment of support and nurturing for the following day.

Classic Interview

Edward Bach was gifted with exceptional intuitive powers which allowed him to simply "know" which Bach Flower essences were the appropriate ones for anyone in any given situation. He realized that not everyone has the same abilities and therefore developed an interview method providing the tools required to prescribe the remedies accurately.

During the classic interview process a trained practitioner guides the person in the selection of the essences to be used. The ultimate goal is to teach the individual how to correctly choose and use the Bach Flower remedies needed without the assistance of a practitioner.

Using this method can be of great benefit; however, one needs to keep in mind that the choice of the appropriate Bach Flower(s) is greatly dependent on the skills, personal perceptions and limitations of the person conducting the interview. The circumstance and personal journey of the interviewer may also inappropriately influence the choice of remedies.

At times we are so overwhelmed with life or find it difficult to truly understand or acknowledge the cause of our challenges, that the guidance of a qualified person is called for.

Conscious Choice

Read about the individual flowers and choose the one(s) you feel are most appropriate for you. You may want to narrow down the choice in the beginning by choosing the appropriate category first. See Chapter 7, *The Seven Categories,* and then continue by reading the individual properties of the flowers within the chosen category.

Example: If dealing with fears, choose that category, read the description for each of the five flowers (*Mimulus, Aspen, Rock Rose, Cherry Plum and Red Chestnut*) and decide which one(s) apply to you.

If you are dealing with a specific mental state or emotion, it is almost like peeling the layers of an onion. First you recognize that you are feeling a certain way, for example you are feeling anxious. The next step is to figure out why you are anxious. If it is because you have difficulties making important decisions *Scleranthus* (Category: Uncertainty) would be indicated. Should your anxiousness be the result of feeling overwhelmed with the responsibilities of life then *Elm* would be the appropriate flower essence from the category of "Despondency and Despair". Maybe you are anxious because you are overly concerned for a loved one which would suggest the use of *Red Chestnut* (Category: Fear).

Using the "conscious" way of choosing the appropriate Bach Flower remedy brings with it some limitations as well. Sometimes it is difficult to be objective; our own perceptions may not lead us to the true cause of the present state of imbalance and disharmony.

Questionnaire

Using a questionnaire can be a useful tool to help find what we need; however, questionnaires have many limitations other than being very time consuming to complete.

Answering questions relies on the conscious mind but, as mentioned before, this may not lead us to the true cause of our situation.

There are many different questionnaires available, each one trying to capture the essence of each Bach Flower in a few words or sentences. The questions reflect to some degree the interpretation of the Bach Flowers of the individual(s) who designed the questionnaire. Some schools/practitioners provide an online questionnaire. Not giving the name of the flowers, you are asked to rate every question on a scale of 1 to 10 (there are 3 questions for every Bach Flower, a total of 117 questions!); the computer will then generate your formula with the five most needed remedies. This sounds like a daunting task and is not very practical when we need instant support or require only short-term help with a situation.

Following are example questions for *Star of Bethlehem* and *Holly* explaining some of the concerns that arise when relying on a questionnaire for the selection of Bach Flowers.

Example Questions from Questionnaires

Star of Bethlehem

- Are you suffering from shock due to bad news or a sudden fright?
- Are you numbed or withdrawn because of traumatic events in your life?
- Have you suffered a loss or grief from which you have never recovered?

The following concerns arise:

- We may not know or be aware of traumatic events in our past because the information might have been withheld from us – intentionally or otherwise.
- We may not realize that a certain event has caused trauma and is affecting us.
- The trauma may have occurred while in the womb.
- We might assume that we have dealt with a loss but in fact the event may still influence us on some level and prevent us from moving forward.

In my practice I have witnessed time and time again how clients burst into tears unexpectedly when talking about some past events. They were convinced that they had dealt with a situation but their reaction was proof of it being otherwise. On some deep level the traumatic experience was still influencing their well-being causing limitations that were unrecognized.

Holly

- Are you jealous, suspicious or filled with hatred for others?
- Are you bad tempered and aggressive?
- Are you suspicious of others, feeling that people have "ulterior motives"?

Sometimes our perception is different from what is really happening or we may not want to admit that these things are within us therefore not answering the questions truthfully or "correctly".

CONCLUSION

Regardless of what method one chooses each one has its advantages as well as drawbacks and limitations. Trust your intuition in the process. Decide for yourself what works best and feels right for you in your individual circumstances. Keep in mind that no harm can be done because *"...the thirty-eight herbs heal gently and surely, and as there are no poisonous plants amongst them there is no fear of ill effects from overdoses or incorrect prescriptions."*–Nora Weeks

HOW MANY FLOWERS TO WORK WITH

*"And with very little effort it becomes
easy to find the remedy or remedies which
a patient needs to help them."*

—EDWARD BACH

Edward Bach's original recommendation was to work with up to six different Bach Flower essences at one time; however, there is no set rule regarding this. The number varies with each situation and depends on the individual. As a general rule I prefer to work with one to four at a time.

Using a greater number of Bach Flowers simultaneously is seldom necessary. Too many may lead to loss or dilution of the focus. People who are more sensitive to all aspects of life may feel overwhelmed and confused with a greater number. The same is true if a person harbours some resistance to personal growth.

Since the idea of working with Bach Flowers is to support a person in bringing them into harmony with their Soul, you want to maximize the effects of the remedies and avoid, or at least reduce, the risk of a person being overwhelmed.

Our level of sensitivity to the effects of the Bach Flowers increases with the simultaneous rise in the vibrational frequencies of the Earth and our physical being, therefore rarely making it necessary to use more than four. There may be the exceptional occasion where more essences are indicated, but typically only in the short term.

The *Rescue Remedy*, consisting of five flower essences, is considered as one remedy.

What to Do if All 38 Seem Right

> *"And now we come to the all-important
> problem, how can we help ourselves?"*

> **—EDWARD BACH**

Sometimes a person does not know where to start and feels like all 38 flowers are needed for support. In these cases it is advisable to enlist the aid of a practitioner or friend who can help narrow down which flowers are needed in the moment and develop a plan of action.

If no support is available, one can work with the issue that seems the most pressing. First think about how you are feeling right now. Next look at the seven categories, choose the one that is most appropriate or you are drawn to, and then narrow down your choice from the flowers in that category.

If you are going through a stage where you feel too overwhelmed or confused and are uncertain of where to start, work with the *Rescue Remedy* for a few days first. Its calming effect will settle things down, making it easier to find the aspect you want to focus on next. Keep peeling the layers of the onion one at a time until you get deeper and deeper and eventually arrive at the core issue.

PREPARATIONS – STOCK BOTTLE AND TREATMENT BOTTLE

Stock bottle: Stock bottles contain a concentration of the Bach Flower essences. They are the ones sold in stores.

Treatment bottle: This is the dilution of the Bach Flower essences prepared for treatments. Treatment bottles hold 25 – 30ml of liquid and the preferred choice are amber glass bottles with a dropper. They might be available at natural food stores, drug stores or pharmacies. Plastic is not recommended because of the chemicals that are likely to contaminate the contents of the treatment bottle. However, if glass bottles are not available plastic bottles serve as a viable option.

Preparing the Treatment Bottle

2 drops from the stock bottle(s) of each Bach Flower essence required is added to a 30ml treatment bottle filled with spring water. In the case of the *Rescue Remedy* 4 drops are added.

Bach recommended the use of spring water, in other words water from natural sources. Many people these days do not have access to clean spring water but fortunately other sources of water can be used instead. If using tap water or well water make sure they are of high quality. Typically tap water contains many chemicals including chlorine and therefore, if it can be avoided, I recommend finding a purer source of water. Filtered water works well as long as it has not been distilled. Distilled water is NOT recommended because it is not "alive" which means it is devoid of vibrations that are required for the transmission of the vibrational frequencies of the flower essences into the water.

STORING BACH FLOWER ESSENCES

No extra precautions are necessary when storing your Bach Flower remedies. They can be kept at room temperature as long as they are not exposed to direct sunlight for extended periods of time.

If there is concern of spoilage a small amount, about one teaspoon, of brandy, cider vinegar or vegetable glycerin can be added to the water. The bottle may also be kept cool in the fridge which for most people is not very practical. These measures are only necessary if the remedy is kept over a longer period of time or in warmer climates.

APPLICATIONS AND DOSAGE

Applications – Internal Use

- Undiluted, straight from the stock bottle
- Diluted from the stock bottle in any liquid (glass, cup or bottle of water, juice, coffee, tea etc.)
- Undiluted from the treatment bottle
- Diluted from the treatment bottle in any liquid (glass, cup or bottle of water, juice, coffee, tea etc.)

In regard to potency and effect of the remedies there is no difference between the diluted and undiluted form taken from either the stock bottle or the treatment bottle. Some claim that the remedies taken straight from the stock bottle have a stronger and more immediate effect. I cannot confirm if this is true.

The efficacy of the remedies is not affected when taken in hot liquid.

Remedies taken straight from the stock bottles have obviously a stronger taste because of the high alcohol content.

Dosage – Internal Use

In my experience counting the drops precisely is not essential for the effectiveness of the treatment. In fact, just like relying on your intuition in choosing the remedy, you can also do the same with the dosage and frequency. Remember the quote from Dr. Bach at the beginning of this chapter to keep things simple.

There is no harm done if taking more drops than the recommended dose, however more drops do not bring faster and better results. In fact, the more sensitive person, the very young and the elderly may do better with a lower dose. It is always better to start with a lower dose. Even though taking Bach Flower essences does not create side-effects like the ones pharmaceutical medications can cause, some individuals may still have a reaction. For more information about this see Chapter 12, *Frequently Asked Questions,* *"What to Expect"* and *"Do Bach Flowers Have Any Side Effects?".*

General Dosage Guidelines

2 drops of each Bach Flower essence when using the stock bottles, or 4 drops of the combination when using a treatment bottle, added to a glass or bottle of water, other liquid or placed directly under the tongue.

The dosage for the Rescue Remedy is 4 drops.

Applications and Dosages – External Use

Diluted or undiluted from the stock bottle or treatment bottle applied directly to the skin. Most beneficial places are the wrists, temples, around the navel, in the hollow at the lower part behind the ears or for those who are familiar with reflexology, the reflex point for the solar plexus on the feet.

In case of physical discomfort the drops may also be applied directly to the affected area.

Skin wash or compress for skin conditions or any other physical concerns: add about 6 drops to ½ litre of water.

Baths – full body, hand or foot baths: add about 2 drops (hand and foot bath) or 5 drops (full body bath) of each Bach Flower essence to the bath water or approximately 10 drops of the treatment bottle.

NOTE: Foot and hand baths are extremely beneficial, gentle yet powerful ways of applying herbal medicines including Bach

Flower essences to the body. The warm water will open the pores of the skin enhancing the absorption of the medicines. In addition, the warm water itself exerts a relaxing and healing effect on the person. Maurice Mességué, a French herbalist, born in 1921, treated people very successfully, using hand and foot baths alone regardless of the condition.

In many countries across the globe people do not have the luxury of a bath tub which makes hand and foot baths a great option. Another alternative is when taking a shower to not allow the water to drain and adding the drops to the water. This way the essences will be absorbed through the soles of the feet.

Spray: the flower essence(s) may also be added to water in a spray bottle and sprayed into the air.

This application will not have a long lasting or very powerful effect but it still works.

For example some of my clients and students have found the spray very beneficial in class room situations where some of the students were extremely disruptive or in meetings that were prone to conflict and dissension.

For some people concern may arise about the ethics of using the Bach Flower essences without the awareness or the consent of people being effected. I believe that Bach Flower essences used as a spray in situations indicated above do not interfere with Soul choice. If a person is not willing or ready to work with a certain issue, the Bach Flower essences will have no effect; so in this sense they cannot override Soul choice. Further, if the remedy is not the one actually needed at that time it will also have no (adverse) effect. Knowing that no harm can be done should erase all concerns. The energy transpiring from the essences only works on positive aspects and helps to create a more harmonious environment.

Many times people use prayer, another form of energy, for

someone without asking permission of the person the prayer is intended for. Energy is also transmitted from our thoughts, our spoken and written words and we do not ask permission when sending out positive or negative thoughts about someone into the universe.

For the very sensitive person it might (initially) be enough to simply have the remedies within close physical proximity, for example carrying them around in a pocket. It may be hard to believe but the Bach Flower essences will exert their effect in this way as well. I have found this to be very useful in cases when the individual is harbouring some resistance or fear of change or personal growth but at the same time on a conscious level has decided to commit to working with the Bach Flowers. This resistance may be on a subconscious level but it is very real. Yet, on a conscious level the individual may have the strong desire to free herself of any limitations that are holding her back from being all who she is. In these cases just being close to the Bach Flower essences may be sufficient before moving on to applying the drops externally and eventually taking them internally.

NOTE: Carrying the Bach Flower essences close to you will eventually not be sufficient to create long-term healing and movement. Other than in the situations described above, this form of application is most effective in challenges that require immediate support and relief and which are of short-term nature only.

The essences themselves will not lose their effectiveness; however, carrying them with you reduces the potential for healing over time compared to taking them internally. Taking the drops internally allows the Bach Flower essence to reach every single cell of the body thus facilitating the "expansion" of all cells, increasing the vibrational frequencies and therefore creating movement and healing, restoring harmony between body and Soul.

Infants are generally very in-tune with the invisible world and demonstrate increased sensitivity to energies. They are very receptive and, like sponges, absorb thoughts, feelings and other forms of vibrations easily without being able to filter "the good from the bad". Applying Bach Flower essences externally may initially be the preferred method of treatment.

Rescue Remedy cream – applied directly to the skin for minor skin irritations. Anyone with sensitive skin may find the cream irritating. In these cases the actual remedies can be diluted in water and used as a skin wash instead.

FREQUENCY AND DURATION

> *"It is then essential to await the result, allowing at least three weeks to elapse before deciding that no benefit has been obtained. If any improvement occurs, no matter how slight, no further dose should be given ... only repeating when the condition becomes definitely stationery, or there is a tendency to relapse."*
>
> —EDWARD BACH

Both frequency and duration depend on the individual as well as individual circumstances. We are all different, reacting to a problem in our own specific way and the same holds true for our reaction to treatment with Bach Flower essences. Frequency and length of treatment need to be adjusted accordingly. As a general guideline the recommended frequency is at least 4 times daily and continued until symptoms subside.

Just like choosing the flowers intuitively, so can the intuition be used as a reliable guide to frequency and duration.

Typically in *acute cases* the diluted or undiluted remedies are taken more frequently over a short period of time, e.g. 4 drops every 5-30 minutes until improvement is noticeable. More sensitive individuals and animals may only require 2 drops. Continue until relief is obtained.

When working with *long-term* situations and prevailing personality characteristics, the recommended dose is 4 drops at least 4 times daily, taken at intervals throughout the day and continued as needed and until you have a clear sense that the essence(s) are no longer required, which may be weeks or even months.

NO IMPROVEMENT after 14 to 21 days? Reconsider the choice of remedies or add different ones.

NOTE: Children are very good in "knowing" for themselves the dosage, frequency and duration for treatment and their judgment can and should be trusted. Since no harm can be done they should be allowed to make their own decision. See Chapter 10, *Who Can Benefit from Bach Flowers – Bach Flowers and Children.*

Frequency and Duration – Examples for Acute Situations

When one of my daughters was sick as a child she would often take half a treatment bottle within two hours and then slow down automatically, sometimes not even finishing the remainder of the remedy.

You come home from work feeling drained and exhausted, physically and mentally, you can take a bath adding a few drops of *Olive* for the exhaustion and add the *Rescue Remedy* if you feel highly stressed. In addition, if you are in need of cleansing because you have dealt with the energy of many people, you might also add *Crab Apple* to help clear the energies.

Frequency and Duration – Examples for Long-Term Situations

You have decided to follow a certain educational path but at times you are lacking interest and thinking of "better things to do", *Clematis* can help you to stay present in the moment.

If lack of focus while studying is the issue, *White Chestnut* will help to clear the mind and make it easier to focus on the task at hand.

Examples for Prevailing Personality Characteristics

The inability to make decisions may require the use of one specific Bach Flower essence over an extended period of time, in this case *Scleranthus*. The remedy may be taken off and on for months or even years and can be considered a central flower accompanying an individual for extended periods of time or even throughout the entire life.

Another example would be someone whose life may be dominated by fear and worrying about the well-being of family and friends. They have the tendency to project negative, disastrous outcomes for the people they feel close to and may interfere with their lives. *Red Chestnut* could be the central Bach Flower essence for this person. Since it is addressing a prevailing personality characteristic *Red Chestnut* may be required for months or years to transform this worry and fear into the ability to care about others in a supportive and calm way and only make themselves available when asked to do so.

CHAPTER 12

Frequently Asked Questions

"Every single person has a life to live, a work to do, a glorious personality, a wonderful individuality."

—EDWARD BACH

WHAT TO EXPECT

"As long as we follow the path laid down by the soul, all is well; and we can further rest that in whatever station of life we are placed, princely or lowly, it contains the lessons and experiences necessary at the moment for our evolution, and gives us the best advantage for the development of ourselves."

—EDWARD BACH

As we take the journey of life as individuals so are our reactions to working with the Bach Flowers specific to our own being.

As you free yourself from limiting beliefs and experiences, you will begin to blossom like a beautiful flower in your own unique way that carries only your signature. This means your experiences and reactions directly reflect your own personal journey of healing spirituality. Reactions may be felt in any aspect of our being – mental, emotional, spiritual and physical.

Recognizing changes of any kind is to some degree dependent on a person's sensitivity, level of awareness and consciousness, where one is in one's life and previous experiences within the energetic realm. It is important to understand that all reactions and changes are perfect, there is no right or wrong way; whatever arrives is perfect for us "right now".

Many people do not have any explicit reactions other than perhaps a general sense of lightness, a feeling of peacefulness, happiness and well-being deep inside. Not all reactions are perceived as positive, someone might feel irritable, restless or easily annoyed by small things. Some individuals are not conscious of any changes or they may not be able to describe or pinpoint them but may simply know that something is different.

Even if you are not aware of anything happening, the spirit of the Bach Flower essence(s) is still working with you, gently flooding your being with its healing and harmonizing light energy. Acknowledge and have faith that whatever is happening is for your benefit, whether you are conscious of any changes or not. If changes are felt they may be recognized immediately, within a few hours, days or not until a few weeks into the treatment.

If no shift is noticed after about two to three weeks, it is useful to reconsider the choice of Bach Flowers; different essences might be needed at this particular time.

Below are some examples of potential reactions and experiences.

FREQUENT REACTIONS

Instant Reactions

- Warmth
- Comfort
- Sense of lightness
- Peacefulness
- Pain (anywhere in the body)
- Softening eyes
- Deep breathing
- Irritability
- Deep sigh
- Joy
- Tingling, often experienced in one part of the body (e.g. the stomach) or on only one side
- Smile, laughter
- Sadness
- Anger
- Tearfulness

Reactions Over Time – Physical

- Old symptoms may flare up
- Symptoms of cleansing (pimples, rashes, increased menstrual bleeding or bowel movements, metallic taste in mouth)
- Skin conditions such as eczema and itchiness (NOTE: On a meta-physical level eczema relates to the suppression of the development of one's personality. The same belief was shared by Rudolf Steiner (1861-1925), founder of anthroposophy. According to Edward Bach

eczema occurs when we do not live our life in accordance
with our Soul.)

- Pain (anywhere in the body)
- Increased or decreased energy levels and vitality
- Increased need/desire to rest
- Muscular tension
- Improved sleep
- Improvement of various physical complaints
- Softening of facial features
- Increased sensitivity of sense organs, for example
  improved hearing and sense of smell

Reactions Over Time – Mental/Emotional

- Feeling cheerful, happy and/or content
- Weight lifted off one's shoulders
- Less or more irritable
- Emotional roller coaster
- Feeling spacey
- Increased patience
- Less aggravated by "small" things
- Hopeful
- Positive
- Sense of clarity
- Easier to talk to and listen to others
- Increased need/desire for alone time
- Increased sensitivity and awareness of nature and need to
  reconnect with the Earth
- Anger
- Anticipation
- Motivation to do things and complete projects

Reactions Over Time – Spiritual

- Increased dream activity
- Activation of energy flow and energy centres (chakras)
- Heightened awareness and consciousness of energies (e.g. sensing of third eye being activated or feeling energy entering through the crown chakra)
- Activation of and trusting one's intuition
- An inner knowing
- Sense of purpose
- Clarity of direction in life
- Seeing/experiencing life in a different, more positive light
- "Sparkling" eyes as the spirit awakens

DO BACH FLOWER REMEDIES HAVE ANY SIDE-EFFECTS?

"As all these remedies are pure and harmless, there is no fear of giving too much or too often, though only the smallest quantities are necessary to act as a dose. Nor can any remedy do harm should it prove not to be the one actually needed for the case."

—EDWARD BACH

Taking Bach Flower essences does not create any side effects in the sense of side effects often experienced when taking pharmaceutical medications. If reactions do occur they are a sign of "movement", of clearing blockages providing opportunities for personal growth. Bach Flowers may stir up situations and emotions from the past that have not been dealt with adequately and therefore on some deep level are still exerting their influence on a person's life in a limiting way.

As the Bach Flower essences fill you with their vibrational frequencies your being is adjusting and learning to harmonize with these higher frequencies. These are exciting times and any experiences and reactions should be acknowledged and embraced as a positive step towards healing.

In the rare event that the reactions are too intense and unpleasant it is advisable to discontinue the use of the chosen Bach Flower essence(s). When you are ready to continue, either work with the same flower essence(s) or choose different ones. If you decide on a new combination, limit the number of flowers to no more than three.

Before taking the essences internally observe your reactions by just having them close by and applying them externally. Provided you are comfortable with this new experience and feel ready, (re) introduce your remedies internally.

CAN BACH FLOWER ESSENCES BE TAKEN ALONGSIDE OTHER THERAPIES INCLUDING MEDICATION?

"This system of healing, which has been Divinely revealed unto us, shows that it is our fears, our cares, our anxieties and such like that open the path to the invasion of illness. Thus by treating our cares, our fears, our worries and so on, we not only free ourselves from illness, but the Herbs given unto us by the Grace of the Creator of all, in addition take away our fears, our worries, and leave us happier and better in ourselves."

—EDWARD BACH

The answer is yes. It is safe to take Bach Flower essences along-side any other form of therapy including conventional medicine and homeopathy. Bach Flower remedies neither affect other forms of medicine adversely nor is the effectiveness of the Bach Flowers influenced by other treatment forms. Many therapies including counseling, psychotherapy and conventional medicine are in fact enhanced when taking Bach Flower essences at the same time.

In my practice I integrate the Bach Flowers with any other form of therapy; they may speed up the healing process and are often the deciding factor in the success of any treatment protocol. One of my students uses Bach Flowers very successfully in her practice when counseling children who have issues as a result of growing up in an abusive environment.

Bach Flower Essences and Homeopathy

Both therapy forms can be combined but it is best not to take the remedies simultaneously.

NOTE: Please do NOT discontinue any medication without consulting with your health care provider first.

DO BACH FLOWER ESSENCES CORRELATE TO SPECIFIC DIS-EASE PROCESSES?

"All know that the same disease may have different effects on different people; it is the effects that need treatment, because they guide to the real cause."
—Edward Bach

There is a lot of information available correlating symptoms and dis-ease processes to specific organs, organ systems and emotions. Traditional Chinese medicine is well known for this concept but it has also become quite popular in recent years in the metaphysical world.

Even though relevant and valid, this system cannot be applied to Bach Flower essences because the remedies do not treat physical symptoms directly. Bach Flower therapy aims at treating mental states and emotions that cause or worsen physical imbalances.

Bach emphasized the importance of thinking first and foremost about a person's current mental and emotional states as well as their personality when selecting the flower essences, disregarding the physical symptoms.

Assigning Bach Flower essences to specific symptoms, dis-ease processes and organs, demonstrates a lack of understanding of how this method works and neglects the importance of an individualized approach for treatment. This applies to the internal and external application of Bach Flower remedies. For example, a book about massage therapy with Bach Flower essences that assigns each Bach Flower to specific skin zones of the body implies that we are all the same. This is fundamentally different from Edward Bach's belief which emphasized that every one of us has our own unique personality fulfilling our own journey on Earth which requires a "custom tailored" approach to healing.

DO I NEED FLOWER ESSENCES THAT ARE NOT PART OF THE BACH FLOWER SYSTEM?

"It is its simplicity, combined with its all-healing effects, that is so wonderful."

—Edward Bach

As a gift of nature rather than a human creation, the system of Bach Flower healing is perfect and complete within itself. It does not require any additional flower essences because Dr. Bach ensured that all possible mental, emotional and spiritual imbalances were being addressed. Even though the Earth is evolving and so are we with it, the emotions we are experiencing now are no different than when Bach lived.

Bach Flowers act on very deep levels, encouraging the individual to take responsibility for their own well-being, facilitating transformation and true healing.

TIMES HAVE CHANGED – ARE THE 38 REMEDIES STILL CURRENT?

"It is as though in this vast civilization of today, a civilization of great stress and strain, the turmoil has been such that we have become too far parted from the true Source of Healing, Our Divinity."

—EDWARD BACH

Even though things have changed drastically from the time of Bach's life in the early 20th century, the emotions and mental states humankind experiences are still the same.

New dis-eases are constantly surfacing but because the Bach Flower remedies do not focus on the physical body but instead address our mental and emotional states, the essences are as current today as they were when the system was first developed.

I believe that the Bach Flower essences might be needed even more today than decades ago. The alienation from nature and from the true meaning of life has become increasingly prevalent with materialism being the dominating focus and aspect in most people's lives. More than ever before we are in need of reconnecting to nature, our spirit, the Higher Self and our Soul for the healing of humankind and the survival of our Mother, the Earth. Bach Flowers can play an important role in bringing us back to these values.

IS IT POSSIBLE TO ACHIEVE PERFECT HEALTH BY TAKING ALL 38 FLOWERS?

I have been asked if we can create perfect health and a perfectly balanced life in harmony with our Soul if we take one course of each of the 38 Bach Flower essences or combine all 38 in one treatment bottle.

Edward Bach had thought himself about combining all 38 Bach Flower essences but found that it did not work. The selection of the accurate remedies according to the personality and emotional state is the best and fastest way to regain balance and get closer to our Soul.

Taking each of the flower essences individually for a specified length of time (one week or several weeks) as a preventative and/or healing measure is not functional. Why for example take *Agrimony* (for mental torment behind a brave face) when it does not apply to our personality or present circumstances? It will have no effect and will not work years in advance should a situation like this arise.

Life presents itself in many mysterious and often unpredictable ways, eliciting various mental states and emotions requiring different skills at different times.

Life is not a constant, it is forever changing and free flowing. So are we growing and changing with every moment and new experience. We come into this life with our definite personality, gifts and purpose but the circumstances we are being exposed to vary and so does the need for specific Bach Flowers.

CAN A PERSON GET DEPENDENT ON OR ADDICTED TO BACH FLOWER ESSENCES?

Bach Flower essences do NOT create any form of dependency or addiction. Once the positive aspects have been established in a person through the increase in vibrational frequencies, the desire or need to continue working with these specific essences will fade away of their own accord. The body will continue to function at higher vibrations without the assistance of the specific remedies. Repeating a specific remedy is only necessary *"when the condition definitely becomes stationary, or there is a tendency to relapse."* (Edward Bach)

ARE BACH FLOWERS SAFE FOR THE ALCOHOLIC TO TAKE?

The amount of alcohol in a single dose is minute, especially when taken from a treatment bottle or further diluted in a glass of water or other drink. If there is concern however, the remedies may be applied externally. For the best effect they should be applied to the wrist, the temples, the navel, in the hollow behind the ears, on the feet at the reflexology point for the solar plexus or at the location of physical discomfort.

Another option is to add the drops to a hot drink allowing the alcohol to evaporate. If you are not comfortable about the safety of taking the Bach Flower remedies, please consult your health care provider.

ARE BACH FLOWER ESSENCES PERISHABLE?

Stock bottles keep indefinitely because they are preserved with alcohol. The expiry date that is currently printed on the packaging and labels of the bottles is due to regulations.

The contents of treatment bottles, if prepared with water alone, will keep for several weeks. Touching the dropper with the fingers or mouth, or keeping the bottle in the heat can cause spoilage before the remedy is used up. In this case the water might turn milky and internal use is no longer recommended. Since the remedy will still carry the vibrational frequencies of the Bach Flower essence(s) it may be safely applied externally, for example in a bath.

Another option is to use them in watering plants or to return them to the Earth.

DOES EXPOSURE TO X-RAYS INFLUENCE THE QUALITY OF BACH FLOWER ESSENCES?

According to research the Bach Flower essences are not negatively affected by x-rays. This means exposure to the scanning equipment at airports will not result in their contamination or reduce their effectiveness.

If anything might affect them it is direct sunlight or heat because both affect the brandy that is being used to preserve the remedies.

CHAPTER 13

How to Get to Know
The Bach Flowers

*"Yet one Truth has mostly been forgotten. That those
Herbs of the field placed for Healing, by comforting,
by soothing, by relieving our cares, our anxieties,
bring us nearer to the Divinity within. And it is that
increase of the Divinity within which heals us."*

—**EDWARD BACH**

Different options are available for deepening your knowledge
and understanding about a particular Bach Flower and there
is no right or wrong way to go about this, it is a matter of individual
preference. Many people have no desire to go into more detail and
wish only to work with the flowers that are appropriate for them at
a given time. The benefits of working with Bach Flower essences are
not dependent on in-depth knowledge of the individual flowers.

However, if you want to familiarize yourself more with these
wondrous flowers, this gift of nature, I suggest the following steps.

STEP-BY-STEP INSTRUCTIONS

Choose the flower you feel most attracted to, or are most curious about at this moment, regardless of why. There is no need to analyze the reason for your choice; getting to know the spirit of the Bach Flowers is best done without engaging our intellect, especially in the beginning.

Another option for deciding which Bach Flower to work with is to focus on a specific question or aspect in your life and choose the Bach Flower that is most appropriate. While practicing one of the exercises described later in this chapter you may ask the spirit of the flower for information and guidance relating to your area of interest.

You might get the impulse to work with more than one Bach Flower, but for the purpose of getting to know the individual flowers on a deeper level, I recommend you only work with one at a time.

Once you have decided on the Bach Flower you want to connect to and communicate with, follow your own intuition or one of the suggestions below.

What to Expect

> *"There are seven beautiful stages in the healing*
> *of disease, these are – PEACE. HOPE. JOY.*
> *FAITH. CERTAINTY. WISDOM. LOVE."*
>
> **—EDWARD BACH**

The results you will receive from these exercises depend to some degree on the attitude with which you approach them. It is important that you open your heart to receiving the information from the Bach Flower essence; it is equally significant that you radiate gratitude and respect, love and sincerity from your heart. When you truly understand and acknowledge that we as human beings are only a small strand in the web of life and that we owe our existence on this Earth to the plant world, the Bach Flowers (as well as all other plants) will share freely with you their spirit and their healing gifts. It is remarkable to experience and even more miraculous that the unconditional love of the plant world continues to blossom and shine, sharing her gifts so freely with anyone who seeks their support despite all the abuse and misunderstanding the Earth has had and continues to endure.

The information and messages you may receive, as well as the way in which they are revealed, will be unique to your own individual being; they may be profound experiences or subtle in nature. Neither one is better than the other, they are all perfect in their own way, helping you to deepen your understanding and awareness of this particular flower while also supporting you on your journey through life.

Some possible experiences of receiving insights might be: dreams, images, sounds, deep inner knowing, messengers from nature (be observant about animals and other signs from nature crossing your path), physical sensations (heat, cold, tingling etc.), tastes, words, heightened sense of awareness, clarity of mind, heightened/increased sensitivity of any or all sense organs, tears, body might vibrate or shake etc.

Accept any sensation and information with an open heart and again, understand that there is no right or wrong way. Regardless of what is happening, you are doing everything correctly as long as you approach any communication with the Bach Flowers with the deepest respect and understanding that they deserve. Sometimes the information may not come to you when you are practicing an exercise but instead at a later time, often when you least expect it. Just remember to keep an open heart and mind, and trust in the process as well as in your own intuition and abilities, and the innate intelligence of the Bach Flowers.

Suggestions

Follow the general guidelines as outlined below for communicating with the Bach Flowers unless you have already developed a method for connecting to plant spirit or your intuition guides you otherwise.

Any of the following practices can be done solely with the intent of deepening your knowledge and understanding of a particular flower or with a question in mind.

General Guidelines for the Practice of Any Type of Exercise

- Take a few deep breaths before beginning an exercise.
- Make a mental note of how your are feeling – physically, emotionally, mentally and spiritually (e.g. pain, sadness, anger, feeling lost or overwhelmed). You may also write your observations down.
- Invite the spirit of the Bach Flower essence to come and reveal itself to you. All you need to do is think about the name of the Bach Flower. If you have an image of the actual flower you might want to have this with you or keep the image in mind.
- At the beginning and end give thanks to the spirit of the flower for being heard and for the willingness to share with you.
- At the end of an exercise "take inventory" about how you

are feeling now compared to before the exercise.

- Journal your experiences and/or share them with a friend, reflect on it, relax and move on with your life.
- Writing and talking about what happened helps to facilitate the movement of the energies, enhancing the effects and creating more potential for healing. Bringing awareness to our experiences through journaling or sharing helps to recognize subtle changes that otherwise might be overlooked easily or taken for granted.
- Continue to observe and be aware of any sensations and changes immediately afterwards and over the next hours and days. Information may come as dreams, insights and ideas, emotional experiences or changes in your physical well-being.

Exercise Options

1. Sit quietly with your eyes closed and be an observer or imagine how the spirit of the Bach Flower fills every cell of your being. As you are doing this be aware of any sensations – emotionally, mentally, spiritually and physically.
   You may ask if the Bach Flower has a message for you. If there is a message it may come as a word or sentence, a sensation, an image, colour, song etc. It depends on how you best communicate with the spirit world.

   When the time is right for completion, thank the flower one more time for coming forward and sharing and when you are ready open your eyes.

2. Read about the flower. Night time is often the easiest time for people to connect with the spirit world because

we are less distracted by outside influences and our conscious mind is less engaged. You may choose to think about the text prior to going to sleep.

3. In the morning journal your dreams or any other note-worthy experiences you might have had. Then read the text again.

4. If you have it available you might take the Bach Flower essence internally throughout the day as well as at bedtime and/or apply it externally. The most sensitive areas to apply the drops to are: temples, in the hollow at the lower part behind the ears, wrists, around the navel and the sole of the feet at the reflexology point for the solar plexus. You may also apply the essence to an area of physical discomfort.

5. Before going to bed, take a bath (full body bath, hand or foot bath) with the Bach Flower essence added to the water.

6. Use the cards from *Bach Flowers Unfolding* to connect to their spirit and support your healing at the same time. See Chapter 16, *Bach Flowers Unfolding* for additional information.

7. Be creative; you may find your own method of connecting with the spirit of the Bach Flower essences that works best for you.

Chapter 14

New Bach Flower Product Developments

"Attempted distortion is a far greater weapon than attempted destruction . . . mankind must always have a choice. As soon as a teacher has given his work to the world, a contorted version of the same must arise – the contortion must be raised for people to be able to choose between the gold and the dross."

—Edward Bach

In recent years new Bach Flower products have been developed and marketed. For example the *Rescue Remedy* can be purchased as chewing gum and pastilles in different flavours. In addition to the *Rescue Remedy* being packaged in various application forms we see new complexes combining specific Bach Flower essences in one formula with the idea to address or treat a specific condition or emotional and mental state; formulas for insomnia, depression, exam anxiety, weight issues or even relationship challenges can be found.

The only premixed formula Edward Bach developed and recommended is the *Rescue Remedy*. This formula is intended as a first-aid remedy for use in a crisis. It addresses the reactions that people typically display in emergencies and it is not intended for long-term use. If required, it is best to follow up with an individualized formula.

It is human nature to constantly find ways to improve life, to make things "better", easier and more convenient. It seems difficult to accept that some things are perfect the way they are, not requiring any changes or "improvements". Great developments and discoveries arise from the desire to search for improvements but this mindset has also caused harm in many areas of life as well.

The healing system of the Bach Flowers was designed by Edward Bach as complete and perfect within itself. The new developments we are seeing are evidence of people misunderstanding, or ignoring the fundamental principles of Dr. Bach's work, the "medicine of the future" as he liked to call it. In his wisdom he anticipated that this was bound to happen.

CONCERNS ABOUT PREMIXED FORMULAS

The development of premixed formulas and other products raises several concerns. Firstly, it is, in my opinion, primarily a marketing strategy and driven by profit considerations. These motives are contrary to Edward Bach's belief and goals in developing this extraordinary system of healing. Bach was inspired throughout his life to fulfill his purpose, serving humanity. Monetary gain was never his interest; in fact he gave up his lucrative medical practice and provided treatments with Bach Flower essences for free.

Secondly, it ignores the most fundamental principles of the Bach Flower system of healing. Bach believed that every one of us is an individual with our very own unique journey through life which requires an individualized approach to healing. No two people are the same which needs to be taken into consideration when choosing a treatment protocol with Bach Flower essences. Key elements in the effective use of Bach Flower essences are: the personality, mental and emotional states, as well as a person's response to a specific situation. All of the above are ignored when formulas are being developed that use the approach of "one size fits all".

Thirdly, developing premixed Bach Flower complexes shows disrespect to Dr. Bach and sadly reflects a lack of understanding of how the Bach Flower system of healing works, as well as its ultimate goal: getting closer to and connecting with our Higher Self so that we may live our life in balance and in harmony with our Soul.

> *"Health exists when there is perfect harmony between Soul and mind and body, and this harmony, and this harmony alone, must be attained before cure can be accomplished."*
>
> —EDWARD BACH

EXAMPLES OF PREMIXED FORMULAS

Rescue Sleep

Rescue Sleep has been developed to enhance a person's sleep and combines the original *Rescue Remedy* with *White Chestnut* to help calm the mind. Granted, for many people this combination might prove to be very beneficial as a symptomatic relief when sleep issues are the result of stress and an overly active mind. However, there are many other circumstances that can manifest in sleep disturbances.

Bach understood that each individual acts and reacts to situations according to their personality, and that different situations can give rise to similar responses in different individuals. This means that even though people present with sleep issues, there are a great variety of situations that can trigger these difficulties and not all of them will respond to the same combination of flowers.

Depression Formula

Depressed emotions can be caused by a great variety of circumstances. A combination of Bach Flower remedies that is aimed at dealing with depression would combine several Bach Flower essences that could potentially be beneficial for this condition. Each one of the Bach Flowers chosen would address a different cause of depression. However, the list of Bach Flowers that relates to depression is long and it is not practical or beneficial to combine all of them into one formula. As a result, a premixed depression formula would only select a few Bach Flower essences that are perceived to address the most common causes of depression, ignoring the specifics pertaining to the individual. It is very unlikely that the formulas developed using the "one size fits all" principle are able to support someone on their healing journey through life in the way Bach had intended.

Following is a partial list of the Bach Flower essences that could be considered for the treatment of depression. Even this partial list includes too many Bach Flower essences to combine into one remedy.

- *Mustard* might be indicated for the person who feels depressed for no apparent reason.
- *Gorse* is the remedy of choice for a person who feels hopeless.

- *Star of Bethlehem* will help to overcome depression caused by grief or a trauma.
- *Elm* is useful if someone is depressed as a result of feeling overwhelmed by responsibility.
- *Larch* might be indicated for the depressed individual who has a lack of faith in their own abilities.
- *Clematis* is for the person who is depressed because they are dreaming of a better future.
- *Honeysuckle* "depression" is caused by longing for or hanging onto the past.
- *Wild Rose* is for the depressed individual who has lost joy in life.

As one can see, there are a great number of "individual" causes for any one condition and the appropriate remedy/remedies should be chosen accordingly.

Exam Formula

You can find an exam formula which includes *Clematis, Elm, Gentian, Larch and White Chestnut.* The idea behind this formulation is to help focus the mind, enhance concentration, calm the nerves and provide confidence.

Although this formula may be beneficial to some it does not allow for individual differences as to why a person might need support in exam situations. For example the above combination does not address any element of fear, a factor commonly associated with exams.

Formulas According to The Seven Categories

I am aware of one company that sells Bach Flower complexes by combining all the flowers belonging to the same category into one formula. For example, the category dealing with aspects of fear includes *Rock Rose, Mimulus, Cherry Plum, Aspen* and *Red Chestnut*; this flower complex will then contain all five flower essences. Presumably this will ensure that any fear, regardless of type and intensity, is being addressed and since no harm can be done, it might be considered a perfect "one size fits all" solution.

The vibrations of each Bach Flower are unique to its own character and mixing them as described above creates density, making each one of them lose some of their light frequencies. It is as though they are bound together in such a way that they cannot radiate and impart their essence freely to the person using them.

True health can only be achieved by using an individualized approach because only then are the Bach Flowers able to connect to us on the deep levels required to create the long-lasting, healing effects of the increase in vibrational frequencies. Any other approach is ineffective.

RESCUE REMEDY PRODUCTS

"Healing with the clean, pure beautiful agents of Nature is surely the one method of all which appeals to most of us, and deep down in our inner self, surely there is something about it that rings true indeed, something which tells us – this is Nature's way and is right."

—EDWARD BACH

The *Rescue Remedy* as developed by Edward Bach was only available in the form of drops. Nowadays it is available as flavoured pastilles, chewing gum, pearls, "liquid melt" capsules and sublingual micro tablets.

Many of these products contain artificial sweeteners and/or other additives. For example the Rescue Pastilles contain artificial sweeteners such as sorbitol.

Bach wished for this new system of healing to be free of impurities. He emphasized the importance of a wholesome diet, close to nature. Are these new products in accord with his wishes, beliefs and principles? I wonder if any alteration from the original ways compromise the quality and effectiveness of the *Rescue Remedy*.

CONCLUSION

I question the ethics behind some of these new developments. The Bach Flower essences, when used as originally intended by Dr. Bach, are able to provide true healing on deep levels of our being by bringing us closer to our Soul through raising our vibrational frequencies. Not adhering to the most fundamental principles in the effective use of these remedies, like losing sight of the importance of taking the personality and the individual response in a given situation into consideration, reduces the potential for personal growth and healing.

Instead of reaching the deep levels of consciousness as originally intended by Bach, premix formulas work symptomatically, something he worked hard to get away from.

Will people using these complexes find relief? Yes, some people will certainly find relief but relief is different than true healing which is the purpose of working with Bach Flower essences.

Unfortunately, our society as a whole is looking for "quick fixes" and prefers to deal with mental and emotional imbalances as well as physical dis-ease in a symptomatic way.

True healing takes courage; the courage and willingness to acknowledge the downfalls and limitations that hinder us from being all we can be and following our Soul's purpose. True healing requires the willingness to take responsibility for our own well-being, which means putting in the effort necessary to make the changes that facilitate growth. True healing involves raising our vibrational frequencies, which brings us closer to the Divine. Ultimately, true healing is only possible when we harmonize our lives with Mother Earth, treat her with the respect she deserves and acknowledge that we owe our existence on this planet to her.

"Healing must come from within ourselves by acknowledging our faults, and harmonizing our being with the Divine Plan."

—EDWARD BACH

CHAPTER 15

Instructions for Creating Bach Flower Essences

"The Earth to nurture the plant: the air from which it feeds: the sun or fire to enable it to impart its power: and water to collect and to be enriched with beneficent, magnetic healing."

—EDWARD BACH

Edward Bach shared his knowledge freely and since his intent was to provide people with effective tools to heal themselves, he made the instructions for the preparation of Bach Flower essences available to anyone.

Preparing Bach Flower essences is easy and can be done by anyone who desires to do so.

MATERIALS NEEDED

- Crystal or glass bowl; do not use stainless steel, aluminum, plastic or oven glassware. Preferably this glass bowl is only used for the creation of (Bach) Flower essences.

- If available, fresh <u>spring water</u> or water from a mountain stream filled in a <u>glass bottle</u>. This is ideal but often not available. In such cases you can also use bottled spring water. Do NOT use city tap water because it is contaminated with chemicals such as chlorine and fluoride. Distilled water should also be avoided because it is "lifeless" and therefore greatly compromised in its ability to absorb the energetic imprint of the flowers; consequently it is limited in passing the vibrational frequencies on to the medicine and its users. Carbonated water is not recommended.

    NOTE: The above recommendations provide for the opportunity to create the purest and most effective Bach Flower remedies possible; however, where none of these sources of water are available it is acceptable to use the kind of water that is obtainable.

- <u>Saucepan</u> for preparing Bach Flower essences with the boiling method. Do NOT use aluminum.
- <u>Scissors</u> for harvesting
- <u>Funnel</u>
- <u>Filtering material</u> such as unbleached coffee filter paper or fine woven, natural material for straining the Bach Flower essence.
- *<u>Glass measuring cup</u> for creating the Mother tincture.
- *<u>Dark glass bottles</u>, 100-500ml size, for bottling the Mother tincture.
- *If available, <u>30 ml amber glass (dropper) bottles</u> for preparation of stock and treatment bottles.
- <u>Brandy, 40%</u> for preserving the remedies. Bach's preferred

choice was brandy because he felt brandy is the purest form of alcohol, however other consumable forms of alcohol are acceptable.

* Whenever available, glass is the preferred choice. Not everyone has access to glassware and in these cases plastic can be used. When using plastic for bottling the final product, the quality and purity of the remedies will be compromised to some degree because some of the plastic components will leach into the essences.

DIRECTIONS – SUN METHOD AND BOILING METHOD

"The process of extracting the healing powers of the plants would thus be simple–as simple as the way in which honey, the most perfect of all foods, is collected from the flowers by the bees."

—Nora Weeks

Preliminary Points to Consider

- Flowers should be harvested on a sunny day and when they are in full bloom.
- Flowers and plants are living beings that respond and communicate in their own unique way with their environment and human beings. An attitude of acknowledgment and understanding, combined with gratitude, respect and love is a prerequisite when harvesting and creating flower essences. This ensures the creation of gentle and most effective remedies, free of contamination from limiting, negative energies. Our thoughts and

feelings can be transmitted into the medicines during harvesting and preparation of the remedies.

- Before beginning to harvest make sure you are in a peaceful state of mind and give thanks to the flowers for their willingness to share their spirit and medicine with us.

Procedure

The following instructions are to be used as guidelines and should be adhered to as closely as possible.

1. Fill glass bowl with spring water and take to the harvesting site.
2. On a sunny day pick enough flowers and other parts of plants required to cover the entire surface of the water. The flowers do not need to be immersed into the water, they can float gently on the surface.

   Care should be taken that the flowers and water are not touched with the fingers. Instead it is recommended to place a leaf of the plant being harvested into one's hand and pick the flowers "with the leaf". If cutting with scissors, the flowers can be cut over the bowl of water and dropped into the water.
3. a) <u>Sun Method</u>

   Let the bowl with the flowers sit in the sun for approximately 3 hours; make sure the bowl remains free of shadows for the entire time. The sun method is used for the more delicate flowers. The first 19 flowers Dr. Bach found plus *White Chestnut* are prepared by the sun method. See below for the list of flowers prepared with the sun method. Bach noticed that the dew drops collected from flowers in the sun were more potent than the ones that had no exposure to the sun.

b) <u>Boiling Method</u>

Boil for ½ hour without a lid, take container outdoors to cool. The boiling method is used for those plants that bloom earlier in the year when there is less sunshine and the sun is not as strong, as well as for those flower essences that require the use of woodier parts. See below for a list of flowers prepared with the boiling method.

4. Take out flowers and other parts, let sediment settle. Do not touch flowers or water with hands.
5. Strain through filter paper into a container – glass, ceramic, stainless steel.
6. Prepare Mother tincture, stock and treatment bottles according to directions below.

PREPARING THE MOTHER TINCTURE, STOCK BOTTLE AND TREATMENT BOTTLE

Preparing The Mother Tincture

Mix equal parts of the "flower essence water" with full strength 40% brandy as a preservative, e.g. 50 ml flower essence water and 50 ml brandy.

Bach preferred to use brandy as he considered it the most appropriate but if necessary you can also use a different form of consumable alcohol at 40%.

<u>Preparing The Stock Bottle</u> (Stock bottles are sold in stores)

Add 2 drops of the mother tincture to 30 ml (1 ounce) of brandy.

<u>Preparing The Treatment Bottle</u>
Add 2 drops of the stock bottle mixture to 30 ml (1 ounce) of
spring water.

BACH FLOWERS PREPARED WITH THE SUN METHOD

*Agrimony, Centaury, Cerato, Chicory, Clematis, Gentian, Gorse,
Heather, Impatiens, Mimulus, Oak, Olive, Rock Rose, Rock
Water, Scleranthus, Vervain, Vine, Water Violet, White Chestnut,
Wild Oat*

BACH FLOWERS PREPARED WITH THE BOILING METHOD

*Aspen, Beech, Cherry Plum, Chestnut Bud, Crab Apple, Elm, Holly,
Honeysuckle, Hornbeam, Larch, Mustard, Pine, Red Chestnut,
Star of Bethlehem, Sweet Chestnut, Walnut, Wild Rose, Willow*

PLANT PARTS USED FOR THE CREATION OF BACH FLOWER ESSENCES

When harvesting the flowers and other parts of the plant used
in the creation of a Bach Flower essence, it is best to pick them
from several plants, bushes or trees.

Agrimony	flowers
Aspen	male and female catkins with a few inches of the twigs and young leaf buds
Beech	male and female flowers, and young shoots with fresh leaves
Centaury	flowering tufts

Cerato	flowers just below calyx
Cherry Plum	flowering twigs
Chestnut Bud	buds with few inches of twigs
Chicory	flowers
Clematis	flowers
Crab Apple	twigs with flower clusters with leaves
Elm	twigs with flower clusters
Gentian	flowers just below calyx
Gorse	flowers
Heather	flowering sprays and leaves
Holly	flowering twigs with female and/or male flowers
Honeysuckle	flowering clusters with several inches of stalks and leaves
Hornbeam	male and female flowers with young twigs and leaves
Impatiens	flowers (only the pale mauve ones)
Larch	male and female flowers with several inches of twigs with young leaf tufts
Mimulus	flowers
Mustard	flower heads
Oak	female catkins
Olive	flower clusters
Pine	young shoots with male and female flowers when male flowers are in full pollen
Red Chestnut	several inches of flowering twigs with young leaves
Rock Rose	flowers
Rock Water	fill glass bowl to top from spring or well

Scleranthus	flowering stems
Star of Bethlehem	flowering stems
Sweet Chestnut	several inches of the twig with leaves, male and female flowers
Vervain	flowering spikes with the least possible number of unopened buds
Vine	flowering clusters
Walnut	young shoot, leaves and female flowers only
Water Violet	flowers
White Chestnut	male and female flowers
Wild Oat	flowering spikelets when in full pollen
Wild Rose	flowers with a short piece of the stem including leaves
Willow	male and female catkins with several inches of the twig with young leaves

NOTE: A practical demonstration of the creation of both the sun and boiling method can be found on the DVD: *Herbal Pharmacy for Everyone – A Step-by-Step Guide to Creating Your Own Herbal Preparations,* available at www.herbalinstructions.com.

CHAPTER 16

Bach Flowers Unfolding
An Innovative Tool for Working
with Bach Flowers

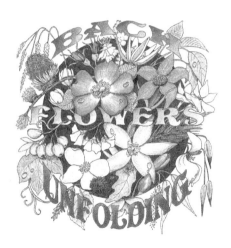

"And as the Creator, in His mercy, has placed certain Divinely-enriched herbs to assist us to our victory, let us seek out these and use them to the best of our ability, to help us climb the mountain of our evolution, until the day when we shall reach the summit of perfection."

—EDWARD BACH

Bach Flowers Unfolding is a unique and practical tool for working with the Bach Flowers. I have created and published this work staying true to the principles of Edward Bach's original work. The essence of the Bach Flowers has also been carefully preserved. I was guided to write *Bach Flowers Unfolding,* adjusting the information brought forth by the Bach Flower essences to the higher vibrational frequencies of the Earth, its elements and humankind. The cards can be used on their own or in addition to the actual Bach Flower essences.

Bach Flowers Unfolding includes a deck of cards, one for each Bach Flower, and a booklet explaining the use of the cards. The booklet also contains information on the use of the actual remedies.

This deck of cards gives detailed descriptions, as presented in this book in Chapter 9, *Detailed Description of the Bach Flowers and Working Guide,* about the respective flower essence in regard to the present state of mind and emotional circumstances a person is experiencing as well as the potentially transformed state. Exquisite full colour illustrations enhance the text.

Bach Flowers Unfolding not only makes deciding which Bach Flower is needed at a given time very easy and practical but it also has other advantages:

- Practical to use for any age group including the very young.
- A lengthy selection process can be by-passed.
- The cards can be used alone or in addition to taking the actual remedies for their healing effect.

   Due to the clarity and intent brought forth during the creation of *Bach Flowers Unfolding* as well as the high vibrational frequencies of both the art and text, each card transmits powerful support and healing. This has been proven time and time again in my practice with clients and students and also by the numerous testimonials and thank you letters I have received over the years.

When I work with Bach Flowers with people in countries such as Mexico, people do not question for a moment the potential healing effect of the cards. This fact is more easily accepted by people whose lives are governed more through their heart rather than the intellect.

- When certain Bach Flowers are only needed short term the cards provide a practical and economical alternative to purchasing the actual remedy either as stock bottle or treatment bottle.
- You can literally "own" and work with all 38 Bach Flowers plus the *Rescue Remedy* without having to purchase the entire kit.
- Easy to take along the whole repertoire when traveling.
- When I travel I always carry a deck of cards with me as support in case I need it. They have proven to be a true life saver in challenging situations.
- For the most sensitive or anyone concerned about the alcohol contents of the essences, the cards provide a great alternative allowing one to experience the benefits of Bach Flowers without taking them internally.

PLEASE NOTE that *Bach Flowers Unfolding* is NOT a replacement for the actual Bach Flower essences. Each form of application of the Bach Flowers has its own characteristic effect on the person and that effect is in part dependent on where a person is on their individual journey in life. Depending on circumstances and the individual, I have seen people achieve more profound healing when working with the cards alone compared to taking the actual remedies. This is true especially in the initial stages of a Bach Flower therapy. It can also be beneficial, for a variety of reasons, to take the Bach Flower essences in conjunction with using the cards.

Taking the Bach Flower essences internally allows the spirit of the flowers to actually "physically touch" each cell of the body, which for many people is necessary in order to receive the full benefit of the potential healing support from the flowers. For these people it seems easier for the body to assimilate the light frequencies of the flowers that create the illumination within that ultimately creates harmony between body, mind and Soul, laying the foundation for healing.

> *"It is a very wonderful thought, but is absolutely true, that certain Herbs, by bringing us solace, bring us closer to our Divinity, and this is shewn again and again in that the sick not only recover from their malady, but in so doing, peace, hope, joy, sympathy and compassion enter into their lives; or if these qualities had been there before, become much increased."*
>
> **—EDWARD BACH**

Both the actual Bach Flower essences as well as the cards from *Bach Flowers Unfolding* are valuable tools that complement each other. They can be used alone or together and their effects depend on each individual. Both are effective.

Bach Flowers Unfolding is available from www.rainbowhealing.ca.

CHAPTER 17

Closing Remarks

*"When we come to the problem of healing, we can understand
that this will have to keep with the times and change
its methods from those of gross materialism to those of a
science founded upon the realities of truth and governed
by the same Divine laws that rule our very natures."*

—**EDWARD BACH**

Edward Bach knew that creating harmony between our
emotions, our mind and our Soul is a prerequisite for a life
lived in happiness and vibrant health. He suggested not to pay
too much attention to our physical body and the actual dis-ease
processes themselves. At the same time he recognized the importance of treating our physical body with good care by providing
proper nutrition, adequate rest and exercise, fresh air and proper
clothing. He also acknowledged that there are times when a
person needs additional support in order to get well.

Many decades have passed since Bach's life in the early 20th century, and even though the emotional and mental states we experience are still the same, the world is changing and has become increasingly polluted with chemicals and toxins. This includes toxins in our food and the environment – the soil, the water and the air, outside and within our homes. Due to advances in technology electromagnetic radiation is of increasing concern to our health and well-being. All of the above put great demand and burden on every one of us. This means that the need to take care of our body on the purely physical level has dramatically increased and is of utmost importance.

We cannot assume that a life lived in mental, emotional and spiritual balance and harmonized with our Soul essence is sufficient to provide long lasting well-being. If we desire good health, we have no choice but to adopt a lifestyle that provides the building blocks for our bodies to continuously renew healthy cells. The basics will be the same for everyone; however, we are born as individuals with specific strengths and weaknesses unique to each one of us, therefore some of us will have to adhere to more rigid guidelines than others. This applies to our physical body and our mental, emotional and spiritual make-up.

Health and healing are very complex and many factors contribute to how we feel at any given moment – physically, mentally, emotionally and spiritually. Being part of a collective consciousness, despite our individuality, we are continuously influenced by everything and everyone around us. We deal with and absorb other people's energies such as thoughts, feelings, and to some degree physical conditions, on a regular basis. Most of the time we are not aware of this happening but nevertheless the transfer of energy is still real and may influence a person's well-being and state of mind to a lesser or larger degree. Bach Flowers can provide support in these circumstances.

The changes in the Earth and the adjustment of humankind to the higher frequencies increases our sensitivity to the interplay of energies now, compared to years ago. As a result, our intuitive senses are (re)awakened and emerge more easily into our consciousness. Our desire to live closer and in harmony with nature is increasing and our experiences with Mother Earth can be more intense and intimate. The effects of this evolution are felt on many different planes and in various ways; the above are only a few examples.

Depending on our personality and journey in life, our response also differs greatly. Thus, in regard to our health, we react as individuals. Some of us are more likely than others to absorb and be influenced by the thoughts and feelings of another person. Health and healing are like a puzzle that consists of many pieces and finding the right piece(s) at a given time is essential, and requires free flowing communication with our Higher Self as well as a connection to our Soul.

> *"Our souls will guide us if we will only listen in every circumstance, every difficulty. The mind and body so directed will pass through life radiating happiness and perfect health."*
> —EDWARD BACH

No matter the situation, Bach Flower essences will lend a helping hand of support and guidance. They can assist us in finding the "right puzzle piece" and may actually be the missing link on our journey to wellness. Bach Flower essences open our channels to the Divine and bring forth light energy, illuminating our being in the most gentle, loving and caring way with any virtue that is required. Their value is as relevant today as it was during the time of Bach's life. In reality, they are perhaps more important and necessary because humanity has strayed even further from the true meaning of life.

Materialistic gain has become the primary focus for most and is the driving force behind a vast majority of developments. The lack of time spent in nature, especially by children, causes behavioural problems and is being described as "Nature Deficit Disorder". Addiction to electronic devices has become a major issue across generations. It is the cause of the break-down in communication on all levels; it alienates us from each other and from nature. We also need to shift our belief system from being the centre of the universe to acknowledging and understanding that humankind is only a small part of the whole and that all other life forms are equal to us, the human race.

In a time of re-awakening, increased consciousness and higher vibrational frequencies, Bach Flowers can play a particularly important role in assisting humankind on its healing journey. True healing requires us to re-connect to nature and to treat the Earth with the respect she deserves as well as returning to values of life that sustain not only ourselves but all life forms on this planet.

"It is in the simple things of life – the simple things because they are nearer the great Truth that real pleasure is to be found."

—EDWARD BACH

Healing of the planet brings with it the simultaneous healing of humankind. This is only possible when we learn to listen to our Higher Self and follow our Soul's guidance which allows us to live our lives harmoniously and with joy in our hearts. Bach Flowers can play an important role and provide great assistance to all in finding their way back to the Truth. Then, and only then, will the planet be healed.

"... it is only when we are happy (which is obeying the commands of our soul) that we can do our best work."

—EDWARD BACH

Bach Flowers are a great tool to guide and support us in achieving balance; balance within ourselves and balance between all life forms and the planet.

May the Bach Flowers accompany you through life like a best friend who is always there for you, filling your heart with joy, listening and responding silently, yet so loud and clear. Learn to trust and understand their guidance so that you may free yourself from limitations and unfold to all of who you are. As the Bach Flowers shine like a guiding star, they can help you transform your life, allowing you to be a shining light yourself, radiating the essence of Love and Truth. In this way you will guide others and give them the courage to do the same. May you receive this gift of HEALING SPIRITUALITY with Love and be Blessed.

DANCING WITH BACH FLOWERS INTO HEALING SPIRITUALITY

Life is like a gigantic and beautiful ocean
It can be calm and still but is always in motion
If the wind is howling and the seas are rough
We might feel lost and feel life is too tough

Remember, our Spirit is here to calm those seas
Working with you silently like busy bees
Creating harmony while illuminating your being
Bringing love, light, hope and healing

Always remember you have what it takes to fly
Just spread your wings and try

You have what it takes to fulfill your dreams
Stay true to your spirit and life will flow like a beautiful stream

Our Spirit is here to guide and support you
in reaching new heights
Giving you courage and all you need
to become a bright shining light
We assist you in keeping open your own Spirit connection
So your life can unfold in most beautiful and
wondrous perfection

May love, peace and hope fill the heart of every single Soul
May tranquil moments bless all and keep our spirits whole
May humankind awaken and create many paradigm shifts
So that all spirits rejoice and undue burdens and challenges lift

Open your heart and you shall receive
The love and light of our spirit indeed
We will lighten your burden and reach deep into your Soul
Sending light into every cell to make life whole

The Earth, our Mother, needs our loving and caring support
Let's reconnect so we may harmonize in accord
May healing of all aspects for all life become true
So our children may have a happy, healthy future too

Let's join our Spirits together
Healing the Earth and ourselves forever
Feeling the joy of dancing happily
To the tune of Healing Spirituality

GUDRUN PENSELIN

Appendix

ALPHABETICAL LIST OF BACH FLOWER NAMES – ENGLISH AND BOTANICAL NAME

Note: In his book, *The Twelve Healers and Other Remedies,* Bach capitalized both, the first and second name of the botanical names of the Bach Flowers. In the official system of the classification of plants, the binomial nomenclature, only the first name is capitalized. In the following list I honor Edward Bach's spelling of the Latin names of the Bach Flowers. Some of the Latin names have been changed since Bach discovered the Bach Flowers. The list gives the currently accepted names.

Agrimony	Agrimonia Eupatoria
Aspen	Populus Tremula
Beech	Fagus Sylvatica
Centaury	Centaurium Umbellatum
Cerato	Ceratostigma Willmottiana
Cherry Plum	Prunus Cerasifera
Chestnut Bud	Aesculus Hippocastanum

Chicory	Cichorium Intybus
Clematis	Clematis Vitalba
Crab Apple	Malus Pumila
Elm	Ulmus Procera
Gentian	Gentiana Amarella
Gorse	Ulex Europaeus
Heather	Calluna Vulgaris
Holly	Ilex Aquifolium
Honeysuckle	Lonicera Caprifolium
Hornbeam	Carpinus Betulus
Impatiens	Impatiens Glandulifera
Larch	Larix Decidua
Mimulus	Mimulus Guttatus
Mustard	Sinapis Arvensis
Oak	Quercus Robur
Olive	Olea Europaea
Pine	Pinus Sylvestris
Red Chestnut	Aesculus Carnea
Rock Rose	Helianthemum Nummularium
Rock Water	
Scleranthus	Scleranthus Annuus
Star of Bethlehem	Ornithogalum Umbellatum
Sweet Chestnut	Castanea Sativa
Vervain	Verbena Officinalis
Vine	Vitis Vinifera
Walnut	Juglans Regia
Water Violet	Hottonia Palustris
White Chestnut	Aesculus Hippocastanum
Wild Oat	Bromus Ramosus
Wild Rose	Rosa Canina
Willow	Salix Vitellina

BACH FLOWER NUMBERS

1	Star of Bethlehem		21	Beech
2	Cerato		22	Gentian
3	Heather		23	Willow
4	White Chestnut		24	Rock Rose
5	Sweet Chestnut		25	Pine
6	Red Chestnut		26	Mimulus
7	Wild Oat		27	Crab Apple
8	Chicory		28	Larch
9	Water Violet		29	Olive
10	Centaury		30	Walnut
11	Holly		31	Rock Water
12	Clematis		32	Chestnut Bud
13	Oak		33	Mustard
14	Agrimony		34	Gorse
15	Elm		35	Vervain
16	Aspen		36	Honeysuckle
17	Wild Rose		37	Hornbeam
18	Impatiens		38	Vine
19	Rescue Remedy		39	Scleranthus
20	Cherry Plum			

Agrimony	14		Crab Apple	27
Aspen	16		Elm	15
Beech	21		Gentian	22
Centaury	10		Gorse	34
Cerato	2		Heather	3
Cherry Plum	20		Holly	11
Chestnut Bud	32		Honeysuckle	36
Chicory	8		Hornbeam	37
Clematis	12		Impatiens	18

Larch	28	Star of Bethlehem	1
Mimulus	26	Sweet Chestnut	5
Mustard	33	Vervain	35
Oak	13	Vine	38
Olive	29	Walnut	30
Pine	25	Water Violet	9
Red Chestnut	6	White Chestnut	4
Rescue Remedy	19	Wild Oat	7
Rock Rose	24	Wild Rose	17
Rock Water	31	Willow	23
Scleranthus	39		

CHART – BACH FLOWERS ACCORDING TO ACUTE, CHRONIC AND SPIRITUAL ASPECTS

During the discovery of the Bach Flowers Edward Bach initially believed that the first 19 flowers he found were specific for acute situations, the following seven would apply to chronic conditions and the last 12 would have their focus on spiritual aspects. He later dismissed this idea.

I have developed the following chart and included it for interest purposes only.

CATEGORY	Acute	Chronic	Spiritual
SENSE OF SECURITY–*Fear*	*Rock Rose* *Mimulus*		*Cherry Plum* *Aspen* *Red Chestnut*
SENSE OF CERTAINTY AND SELF WORTH AS A RESULT OF TRUST IN INNER KNOWING – *Uncertainty*	*Cerato* *Scleranthus* *Gentian*	*Gorse* *Wild Oat*	*Hornbeam*
STAYING FOCUSED IN THE PRESENT IN ALL THAT YOU KNOW – *Insufficient interest in present circumstances*	*Clematis*	*Olive*	*Honeysuckle* *Wild Rose* *White Chestnut* *Mustard* *Chestnut Bud*
NURTURE AND SUPPORT SENSE OF TRUST AND BELONGING – *Loneliness*	*Impatiens* *Water Violet*	*Heather*	
STRENGTH TO STAY FOCUSED AND TRUE TO ONE'S OWN IDEALS – *Over-sensitivity to influences and ideas from others*	*Centaury* *Agrimony*		*Walnut* *Holly*

CATEGORY	Acute	Chronic	Spiritual
ENCOURAGEMENT AND CONTENTMENT WITH HEIGHTENED SPIRITUAL KNOWLEDGE – *Despondency and despair*		*Oak*	*Crab Apple* *Elm* *Larch* *Pine* *Star of Bethlehem* *Sweet Chestnut* *Willow*
LIVING IN SYNCHRONIZED BALANCE AND UNDERSTANDING OF THE HIGHEST (HEART WOVEN) TRUTH – *Over-care for welfare of others*	*Chicory* *Vervain*	*Rock Water* *Vine*	*Beech*

BIBLIOGRAPHY

The Bach Flower Remedies. New Canaan, Connecticut: Keats, 1979.

Includes *Heal Thyself* and *The Twelve Healers And Other Remedies* by Edward Bach and *The Bach Remedies Repertory* by F.J. Wheeler.

The Work of Dr Edward Bach. An Introduction and Guide to the 38 Flower Remedies. London, England:Wigmore Publications Ltd., 1997.

Howard, Judy. *Growing Up With Bach Flower Remedies.* 3rd edition. Saffron Walden, England: Daniel, 2008.

Howard, Judy, and John Ramsell. *The Original Writings by Edward Bach.* Saffron Walden, England: Daniel, 1990.

Mességué, Maurice. *Of People & Plants. The Autobiography of Europe's Most Celebrated Herbal Healer.* Rochester, Vermont, USA: Healing Arts Press, 1991.

Penselin, Gudrun. *Bach Flowers Unfolding.* Wembley, Alberta, Canada: Rainbow Healing Publishing, 1998.

Scheffer, Mechthild. *The Encyclopedia of Bach Flower Therapy.* Rochester, Vermont, USA: Healing Arts Press, 2001

Weeks, Nora. *The Medical Discoveries of Edward Bach Physician.* Saffron Walden, England: Daniel, 1991.

Weeks, Nora, and Victor Bullen. *The Bach Flower Remedies. Illustrations and Preparations.* Saffron Walden, England: Daniel, 1990.

VIDEOS

Bach Flower Remedies – A Further Understanding. The Dr. Edward Bach Centre 1992.

Herbal Pharmacy for Everyone. A Step-by-Step Guide to Creating Your Own Herbal Preparations. Instructional DVD. Gudrun Penselin 2012.

The Light That Never Goes Out. The Dr. Edward Bach Centre 1992.

RESOURCES AND RECOMMENDED READING

Ball, Stefan, and Judy Ramsell Howard. *Bach Flower Remedies for Animals.*

Ball, Stefan, and Judy Ramsell Howard. *Emotional Healing for Cats.*

Ball, Stefan, and Heather Simpson and Judy Ramsell Howard. *Emotional Healing for Horses and Ponies.*

Chancellor, Philipp M. *Illustrated Handbook of the Bach Remedies.*

Howard, Judy. *The Bach Flower Remedies Step by Step.*

Müller, Beatrice C. And Siegfried Koepfer. *Blütenbilder – Seelenbilder.*

Scheffer, Mechthild. *Bach Flower Therapy. Theory und Practice.*

Wheeler, F.J. *The Bach Remedies Repertory.*

WEBSITES

- Dr. Edward Bach Centre/Dr. Edward Bach Foundation, Sotwell, Wallinford, England.
  www.bachcentre.com

- Flower Essence Services, Nevada City, California.
  www.fesflowers.com

- Nelson Bach USA, Wilmington, MA.
  www.nelsonbach.com

BACH FLOWER
REFERENCE INDEX

———————————

GUDRUN PENSELIN

"I see her (Gudrun) as a healer and friend to those around her and the Earth itself, and am constantly inspired to strengthen my own commitment to living a life based in Love... and the singular dedication to the much needed healing of the Earth and its people."

—**LANA ROBINSON, B.A.,** Presiding Clerk of Canadian Friends Service Committee (CFSC)

Gudrun Penselin, M.Ed., is an author, speaker and expert in herbal medicine. She often conducts workshops on herbal pharmacy, connecting to plant spirit, reflexology, light and colour therapy, lifestyle improvement and, of course, the Bach Flowers.

Gudrun has written articles on several topics including medicine making with dried herbs, using Wild Rose and Rosehips for food and medicine, encouraging healing with Bach Flowers, and connecting to the Earth. She is the executive producer and co-creator of the instructional DVD *Herbal Pharmacy for*

243

Everyone, A Step-by-Step Guide to Creating Your Own Herbal Preparations and created the *Bach Flowers Unfolding* card deck.

Gudrun is a natural educator who brings joy whenever she shares her knowledge and experience about plants and their healing spirit. She is a frequent presenter at conferences in Canada and the US and has been a featured guest on numerous radio shows.

Gudrun was born and raised in Germany. Since her emigration to Canada in 1981, she has focused her professional education on complementary medicine. For over 30 years she has been running a successful practice in Grande Prairie, Alberta. She has helped thousands of people through her teachings and practice by using a holistic approach to wellness.

She enjoys the outdoors and being close to nature. Gudrun has explored many parts of Canada with her family while camping, canoeing and hiking in the wilderness. Her deep interest in learning about other cultures and their healing traditions led her to travel to many places across the globe, including India, where she was fortunate to spend some time with Mother Teresa. More recently, her travels have taken her to Central and South America, where she focused her attention on some of the traditional forms of healing.

Gudrun Penselin, M.Ed., M.Phys.Ed.
Clinical Herbal Therapist, Bach Flower Practitioner,
Certified Reflexologist, Certified Iridologist/Sclerologist,
Light/Colour Therapist

For more information about Gudrun's work, visit
www.rainbowhealing.ca and www.herbalinstructions.com

CPSIA information can be obtained
at www.ICGtesting.com
Printed in the USA
FSOW04n0822190517
34213FS